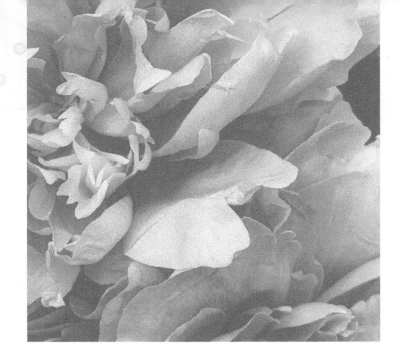

WELCOME
to your journey

Hey, there I just want you to know that
YOU. GOT. THIS!

Acknowledgments

I am immensely grateful to everyone who contributed to the creation of this book. Writing and publishing have been transformative experiences, and they would not have been possible without the encouragement and support of many.

To my family, especially my children Joanna, Yael, Enoch, Micah, and Eden, thank you for your encouragement and patience through the long days and nights spent writing. You all are the reason I keep moving forward even through discouraging and hard times. I love you more than words.

I thank God for the Inspiration and desire to embark on this project even when it felt bigger than me.

Closing Remarks

To everyone who touched this project, from the early drafts to the final product, your contributions have been immeasurable. Thank you for being part of this journey.

TABLE OF CONTENTS

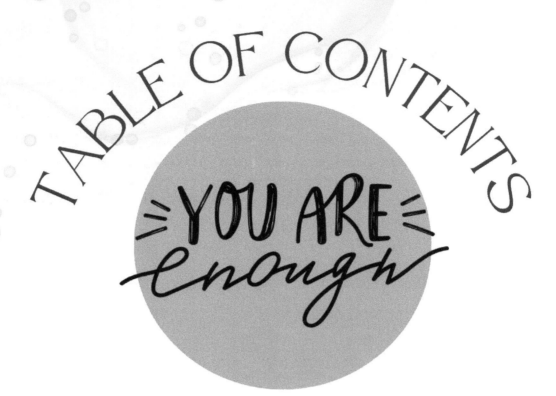

YOU ARE enough

CHECK-IN

LIST THE TOP 12 WORDS THAT DESCRIBE YOU

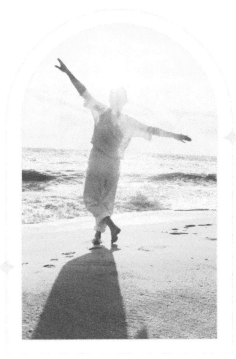

HEY THERE!

Write Out What you Hope to Get From This Book

If you would like the support of experts and a community of like-minded women during your transformation, then check out the 12-week online program at www.EverydayNurse.com

DEAR _____

(your name)

It's time for you to feel like yourself again.
It's always been time.

You are made for more than you have dared to believe lately. I know you have felt tired, anxious, and even overwhelmed. Becoming you again has seemed distant and maybe even scary, and that's why I am here. I want to show you that your true identity, the parts of you that bring you the most joy and peace, are wrapped up in love. Love that flows from you, and love that flows to you in the present from the ultimate source, God. Your past has taken up enough space in your life, leaving you stagnant and dissatisfied and feeling like a stranger in your own life.

I know you were once a little girl full of dreams, promise, belief, and hope, and you were set to change the world. Then someone came along, and either through words or experiences, made you believe your dreams were too dreamy. Slowly, your dreams were stolen, and your identity was replaced by self-doubt. Something changed when life did not show up how you expected it would, and you stopped looking for the beauty in your present and instead have chosen to with a desire to replay the past.

If you peel back the negative thought patterns and adjust the flashlight to shine forward rather than into your past, you will discover so much beauty, so much of you still thriving and hungry for life. You will see a beautiful future defined by who you have become, a lovely butterfly surrounded by fragrant relationships while painting the world with your beauty.

If you are having trouble believing what I am saying, I understand. I've been there, too, and many other women have. But I am forever thankful that someone helped me see myself again and helped me believe that there was more in me, infinitely more, because God's Spirit is within me, An endless source of love.

God wants you to have life and to have it more abundantly.
(John 10:10)

♥ – Annie Chitate

PREFACE

I remember the first time I thought about health differently. My firstborn was about seven months old, and she was having a hard time with teething. I felt like it really hurt, and as her mother, I wanted to do anything to have the pain myself and watch her run around and play freely. The options I had at the time were giving her a cold thing to chew on, a teething toy, applying the gum creams, etc, as well as giving her some popular children's pain medication and watching the pain melt away. And that's where my struggle began. With all the side effects that I had memorized and rehearsed as a nurse, there was a war within my mind. Where does it stop? How many times am I going to have to medicate her before the end of this teething cycle? And what about the rest of her teeth, which will also have to erupt?

That day, I had a tough time because it was the first time I had not just reflexively given medications. In the hospital, I sometimes felt like a med-passing robot, and I just handed them out as prescribed, making sure to tell the patients what the potential side effects were. Even though some of the side effects promised were worse than their current illness, we humans like quick solutions, and we hope for the best outcome in the future, even when we aren't working towards it. So here I was on Google, looking for alternatives and feeling like a sell-out to my training and my passion as a nurse. I love and respect the role nurses fill in the health field, and if most people knew what nurses go through daily, we would be giving them hugs whenever we see them... and, of course, a good old pay raise! ... But back to the Google search, I was faced with so many random suggestions of what I could do to alleviate my child's teething pain. After a good, overwhelming 5 minutes, I closed the computer, headed to her father, and pitched a random suggestion to get trained in holistic wellness.

Fast forward a year and a half, and we found ourselves at the most beautiful little campus in Colorado, a wellness center, learning things that had us, as nurses, constantly checking the science; it was almost unbelievable! We were learning how to treat our body holistically, as one machine, and seek out the cause of our symptoms instead of covering them up with medications. We watched people come for two weeks and leave without type 2 diabetes (a lot of them stopped needing their medications by day 5), High Blood Pressure, Anxiety, Insomnia, and many other lifestyle diseases.

I watched as people lost tens of pounds in those two weeks, tumors began to shrink, and a lady who had come in with heart failure was taken off the heart transplant list by her doctor because she had started getting better after two weeks of the experience. It was just mind-blowing, and I was sold!

I started learning a lot about children's remedies and, more importantly, how to live a healthier life so that we could be happier, more productive, and more fulfilled. Even with all that incredible stuff, I still remember the day my life truly changed for the better. A lady named Barabara O'Neill came to teach for two weeks, and I had never heard health explained so simply and clearly as I did sitting in her lectures. It was through her lectures that I came to realize that I had a hormonal imbalance. All those symptoms or feeling `unwell" vague symptoms and things other people would raise an eyebrow to start to make sense. I listened and started implementing the things I learned. What do you know? I began to see results.

Soon, I began to get questions from family and friends whenever they had symptoms or their children were sick. They wanted to know what they could do at home if it weren't severe enough to go to the doctor. They also wanted to know what might have caused the illness so we would do assessments, look at the gaps in their lifestyle, and pinpoint the source of the issue. Sometimes, it was diet; other times, it was lack of movement, stress from life or emotional chaos, and other sources. This is not to say that people are not genetically prone to certain illnesses, but as the great quote by Caldwell Esselstyn says, "Genetics load the gun, but lifestyle pulls the trigger." Being genetically prone to something like type 2 diabetes does not automatically give you type 2 diabetes; the conditions under which it becomes expressed have to be a part of your lifestyle, i.e., all the possible triggers of type 2 diabetes that can be found in the American diabetes association website or the World Health Organization information on the disease.

Since then, I have run international women's groups on wellness, specializing in mothers' and children's health, held presentations on the topic, and done one-on-one consultations to help many women find freedom for their pain points. The most significant tools that have given me much success and helped me understand women are having gone through the journey myself, seeking better health for myself and my children, and my extensive knowledge from my training as a nurse.

Having an understanding of the human body from a biological perspective is a reason I believe Barbara O'neill's presentations are so fantastic. She, too, was trained and worked as a nurse before learning about natural health over 40 years ago! That training has also helped me to simply re-route some of the women who have come to me to the hospital. Some symptoms may be orange or red flags, and though a person may want to apply natural means to it, they may need medical help right away. Once the acute situation is stabilized, they may look into natural methods to help them along. A good example of this would be someone having a hypertensive crisis where their blood pressure is so incredibly high that they need to go to the emergency room right away and allow the caring nurses and doctors to nurse them to stability. Once they come back home, they can make the necessary changes to ensure their blood pressure gets back to normal levels and stays there, and they never have to experience that life-threatening condition again!

In the last few years, a few women have encouraged me to make this simple yet profound information available to more women; it's pretty mind-blowing how sensible it all sounds and how effective it is when they try it. At first, I resisted because it seemed like a vast tall mountain, and I listened to the self-doubt that said... but there are already others teaching this; I can sit in my comfort zone; why would anyone hear what I have to say? I'm glad I ignored the negativity because you needed to hear this, and I needed to hear it again. If Barbara O'neill had listened to those voices of doubt, I wouldn't have had the opportunity to sit in her lectures and change my family's legacy. So I listened to the call, and that's when I founded Everyday Nurse, a platform dedicated to women's holistic wellness. I then collaborated with some amazing experts, and we created a transformational experience that is wrapped up in a 12-week program and we march together like a victorious army, leaving no one behind. This book was also born out of that desire to bring help to those who may want to make an individual journey to transformation. Yes, it has been a lot of work, but sharing my story has been well worth it.

The same applies to you; there is a calling inside you today. It has existed for a while and sometimes feels dried up. I'm here to sprinkle some life-giving water on it and let it be rehydrated as your health blossoms. You are coming alive, lady; I know you already feel it, and even as I write this, I'm smiling and tearing up simultaneously because I know what it's like to feel stuck and then come alive. YOU. CAN. DO. THIS!

Cheers to your health, which is exceptionally greater than wealth... cheers to you!

Step One

Emotional Access

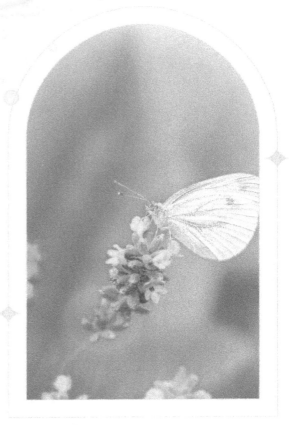

Wellness, like motherhood, is not a destination but a journey—a delicate balance of harmony and chaos directed by the chemical waves of our hormones.

WEEK 1
Believe In Tomorrow

I was homeschooling my six-year-old son one day when I asked him to go to the little blackboard we thrifted and write a word that I knew was a little harder than he was used to. This little guy has the most pleasant, happy-go-lucky attitude, dark, long lashes, and an easy smile that lights up everyone he shares it with. But this day, his head swung my way with a big open gasp as he said, "I can't do that; it's too hard!". I was steady with a tender smile and with eyes full of confidence as I said in a soft, firm tone, "Yes, son, you can! Just sound it out like the other words and write what you hear". I was confident he could do it! I just wanted him to know he could. He wanted to believe this grand belief I had placed in him, so he shuffled his feet to the board and turned to look at me as if to question me one last time before he started to sound out the word and write it down. Soon, I saw a smile break his lips again because he began to see what I knew all along. He was doing it!

As women, there are many areas in our lives where our beliefs are not based on the truth. How we feel about our bodies, our lives, our achievements, and how we feel about our motherhood or contribution to our jobs and society. These thoughts are often based on our perception and not truth. Our thoughts are a collection of words, and often time the words that stand out are those collected from negative interactions, mistakes, and failures. If we are not intentionally fighting the gravity of our thought patterns, we find ourselves in slumps and cannot even recall how we got there. After a while, we begin to find it hard to believe anything positive people say about us... Pure drops of kind words and compliments often roll off our backs, oiled with self-doubt and negative talk.

You may be in such a space right now; I sure was. For years, I did not believe anything good was left for me. I believed the saying "the best days are behind you," and I lived it out, only tolerating the present and looking back to the days when I was beautiful, smart, desirable, and relevant. Isnt it sad that we believe the cookie-cutter lies. There is no truth in any of it.

It may be true that you've had rough patches and life played out differently than you thought it should. It certainly has for me, and I spent years in the prison of depression. But I want you to look around you with a different lens for a minute, think of how resilient you are, how wise you have become, and how brave you must be to desire better, or you would not be reading this book. Something great has been happening in you through your experiences, no matter how painful they have been.

WEEK 1

A while ago, I heard someone say that 'we only see what we focus on', and I had to pause. Could it be that I have only seen sorrow and pain, crumbling dreams and hopelessness because those are the things I was focused on? It was hard for me to accept that there was anything else but that in my life. I felt powerless. But that statement offended me, and then, after a while, it challenged me just to consider the possibility that there was more to my story. After all, "there is no such thing as a one-sided coin" - Myron Golden. I want to present the same challenge to you. On the other side of every negative thought and feeling is a positive one. Practice turning over the coin and allowing yourself to be amazed at the positivity and value you will see there. I realized that I had grown during the hard times; I was different, wiser, and more valuable, and my gifts had been expanded. I want to challenge you to shift your focus, seek out the good, seek out your true self, the beautiful creation that you are.

You are beautiful. Yes, you are. Say it. You are a joy to be around. You are a good mother. You are doing the best you can with the tools you have. You have a place in this world, that dream that has not yet been realized.

I want to give you room to grow your knowledge of the truth about yourself. I want to give you access to people who will cheer for you, encourage you, and lovingly remind you that you can be happy and whole again.

Everything we say about any future outcome is just a belief. There are no facts involved. When you hear someone say, " UGH! Mondays are the worst," that's absolutely untrue. Some of the best days of your life have been Mondays, just as equally as Tuesdays and Fridays. But we have decided to frame Mondays in a negative light, and that often leads to us seeing everything that happens on a Monday through a negative lens. Our brain is created to make us the hero, so if we say it, it must become true as much as possible. If I started saying my favorite day is Monday, I would begin to zoom into the positive aspects of Mondays and enjoy every single Monday: why? Because my brain is biased toward my opinion, it will highlight whatever helps me feel like I'm right!

So, it is extremely important for us to only speak positive thoughts and conclusions about our future outcomes, our bodies, our children and even our past!

My past happened for my good! It is up to me to accept that good.

What does this have to do with your hormones? Everything! Your body is an incredible circle; every minute of every day, blood full of nutrition and oxygen and chemical messengers travel around the circle, from the heart to the brain, to the body, and back again. The messengers report any pain, strain, fatigue, or happiness, and the Message echoes through the entire body so that pain in your toe from accidentally kicking the corner of the doorpost can make your head hurt and make you want to sit down, you may also groan or scream and your breathing changes. All those changes happen because the entire system is affected by the pain in your toes.

Emotional pain works the same way; it echos through your body, causing physical changes throughout the system. No matter how much physical work you do to get your life and health on track, if you don't first resolve your mental pains and correct your mindset, you will find yourself chasing the wind because nothing physical can cure a broken spirit.

I'd like your permission to walk with you on this journey to get your mind whole.

The next two weeks will be focused on helping you access the feelings and thought processes that are not serving you. You will have to uproot them and throw them in the trash! Then, we can revive the truth about who you are and who you were created to be and revive your unique calling. See, I will not be the one to tell you those truths because I did not create you. Only your Creator can fill you with truth, and He will if you allow it.

As you explore what you believe about yourself in your core, I encourage you to be vulnerable and allow yourself access to the truth. I know you can do this! And if you are unsure, lean on my beliefs until yours grows. YOU. GOT. THIS.

Day one

List 3 negative thoughts you have believed about yourself

_____

_____

_____

_____

Can you recall any specific sources for these thought patterns?

_____

_____

_____

_____

_____

For each negative belief, write down one instance when it was not true. (for example, if you feel like you are a mean person, think of a time you were kind)

_____

_____

_____

_____

_____

_____

_____

MOOD (FEEL)

😊 😌 😐 😟 😢 😬 😑

REFRAME: Using the answers above, make a positive statement, say out loud " I am a kind person because I helped the old lady cross the road last fall)

Day two

Identify 5 ways you believe you have changed in the last 10 years

_____

_____

_____

_____

_____

_____

Describe the reasons you believe those changes happened

_____

_____

_____

_____

_____

_____

_____

_____

Do you feel like you have control over the things that happen in your life? If not, why not?

_____

_____

_____

MOOD (FEEL)

_____

😊 😌 🙂 ☹️ 😢 😬 😐

Day Three

Picture your ideal self: write down everything about her, including how she looks, her lifestyle, her emotional state, and how her close relationships feel.

_____

_____

_____

_____

_____

_____

_____

_____

_____

_____

_____

_____

_____

_____

_____

Whats the ONE thing stopping you from being that person?

_____

_____

_____

MOOD (FEEL)

☺ ☺ ☺ ☹ ☹ ☺ ☹

Remember, you are the CEO of your life and you always have power to determine what your future looks

Day Four

Write a letter to yourself, forgiving yourself for decisions you have made that you regret. I would like you to be very specific. (If your letter contains personal information that you feel someone may access in this journal, write it on a separate piece of paper that you can shred or burn). At the end of the letter, express Love, understanding, and gratitude to your past self because those decisions made you who you are today.

Dear ....I forgive you for

_____

_____

_____

_____

_____

_____

_____

_____

_____

_____

_____

_____

_____

_____

_____

_____

_____

MOOD (FEEL)

_____

Day Five

Think of 10 things you believe you were created for. These could be relational, creative, or productive.

_____

_____

_____

_____

_____

_____

_____

_____

_____

_____

_____

_____

Which of the ten inspires you the most, and why?

_____

_____

_____

_____

_____

_____

MOOD (FEEL)

_____

Day Six

During yesterday's exercise, you listed ten things you were created for. Pick 3 things from the list and write how you are currently living out your purpose in those 3 ways.

_____

_____

_____

_____

_____

_____

_____

_____

_____

_____

_____

_____

_____

Please write down your favorite quote or verse and explain why it inspires you.

_____

_____

_____

_____

_____

MOOD (FEEL)

☺ ☺ ☺ ☹ ☹ ☺ ☺

Day Seven

Write a letter to yourself from the perspective of your best friend, mother, sister, husband, or whoever you are closest to. Write the letter as a letter of appreciation, listing all the great things the person enjoys about you.

MOOD (FEEL)

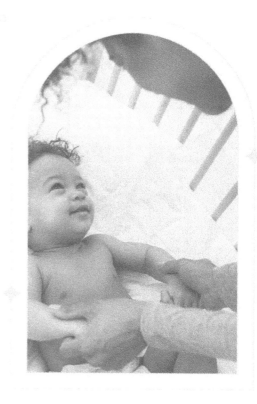

Motherhood is not a test but a journey. It's not about how much you do or how well you do it, but about the love you give and the moments you share."

WEEK 2
Embracing Positivity

A fascinating story is told in the Bible of a king named Jehoshaphat and a battle he faced against an incredibly strong and vast army. This king was humble enough to know he could not win against them and wise enough to know he needed help much stronger than himself. So he prayed and called everyone to fast with him. He received the most incredible response from God, who said, " Don't be afraid of this vast army; I'll fight this battle for you." Let's just pause there; I want you to imagine the one thing you would do if you absolutely knew you'd succeed. Maybe, like me, you have one thousand and twenty-seven things you would do. Imagine the focus you would apply to those things. You would put 100% of yourself into that thing and start right away, wouldn't you?

Ok, let's get back to the story. So Jehoshaphat made one of the most unusual and bizarre battle moves in history; he called the musicians and had them lead the army into battle! As they arrived at the battle site, singing songs of gratitude and praise for their future win, they realized that the battle was already fought and won. Their enemies, a group of powerful kings, had turned against each other, and all King Jehoshaphat and his army (and choir) had to do was collect the treasures these men had left behind. PAYDAY!

Again, I ask you, what would you do if you had guaranteed success? Would you work on certain relationships in your life? Maybe it's that business or financial goal that you have felt is far out of reach, or would you mother differently? How about on the inside? What habits, character qualities, and thought patterns would you want to adopt if you knew you would SURELY succeed?

Becoming is a process more guaranteed than we often think. The common thought is that life happens to us, and we just receive whatever it throws at us. A huge part of accepting that mindset is our general desire to escape the reality of our choices in the cause-and-effect equation. Now, I know some horrible things may have happened to you that you had ZERO control over, and you may need to talk to a professional and get the tools you need to mentally process those life events and begin your journey to healing. However, in this chapter, we will be processing our daily action-reaction experiences.

Life can often be likened to a garden experience of sowing and reaping. Today presents an opportunity to sow tomorrow's feelings of joy or regret. The only thing that has stopped you from sure success in the past has been a lack of awareness of the Jehoshaphat-like promises available to you. Prepare to grow your winning mindset when it comes to overall wellness, as this is the focus of our journey together.

WEEK 2

In the previous chapter, we dealt with limiting beliefs and how to reframe them. But during this part of our journey, we are addressing your current battles. You may be facing financial, relational, or health challenges, or you may have anxiety that has set in. Perhaps you have picked up some negative coping mechanisms that you felt could help you get by, but these have just added to the forces against you. It's easy for us to feel overpowered by the battles when all we desire is freedom.

The freedom to be happy, whole, and live a life of purpose and fulfillment comes at a cost. You have to be willing to fight for it.

Are you willing to fight? Say out loud, "I AM WILLING TO FIGHT." You are sowing seeds for a new and beautiful future. Remember the power of words. When you say it, your mind works with you to prove it.

I am very proud of you for being willing to fight. You will win.

Often, we believe that joy and peace will come when the struggle is over. But how many of us know of people who reached the end of their lives and never found peace? Peace and joy are not the result of achieving wealth, status, or trending standards of beauty. I have seen too many people who seem to have achieved all of the above life on mind-altering chemicals or even take their own lives because Peace and joy are not achieved; they are received. Let that sink in. They are available to you right now in your present circumstances.

The simplest concepts can be the hardest to accept. A common illustration shares the power of perspective.

"Once upon a time, in a small village in rural China, an old farmer worked his crops for many years. One day, his horse ran away. Upon hearing the news, his neighbors came to visit. "Such bad luck," they said sympathetically. "Maybe," the farmer replied.

The next morning, the horse returned, bringing with it three other wild horses. "How

wonderful," the neighbors exclaimed. "Maybe," replied the old man. The following day, his son tried to ride one of the untamed horses, but he was thrown off and broke his leg. The neighbors again came to offer their sympathy for his misfortune. "Maybe," answered the farmer.

The day after, military officials came to the village to draft young men into the army. Seeing that the son's leg was broken, they passed him by. The neighbors congratulated the farmer on how well things had turned out. "Maybe," said the farmer.

WEEK 2

I think you can see that all it takes is a different perspective to change your feelings about past or present circumstances.

Joy is a result of the words you assign to your story. The words in your mind and the words out of your lips. You have ALL the power to give joy or take it away, both for yourself and those around you. You can choose to put on positive lenses and consider, even for a moment, that every circumstance can turn out very positively and work out for your good if you let it. At first, you might feel uneasy, and you may even face some internal hesitation accepting this, but look around you and see people who are where you would like to be, how many of them have humble or even difficult beginnings. No one is exempt from negative experiences, but we all get to choose how we react to them and who we become from them.

Joy is something you can choose today through gratitude.

When you are grateful for everything, you choose to view your circumstance from the lens of a positive outcome, no matter how it began and is going. Sometimes, it is hard to be thankful while you are in what seems to be a fiery pit, but that fire is purifying the gold in you. Practicing daily gratitude will almost instantly change your lens and give you the gift of peace.

Peace is simply the result of recognizing that God is that kind and tender parent who can help you clean the mess, fix the broken toy, or replace it. He will put food on the table and keep you clothed and sheltered. All you have to do is give Him permission to do so, let him have the leadership of your life, and just like children do not stay up at night worrying about stuff, you can sleep in peace. Peace is assurance, not in yourself cause clearly... need I say more?...but in One who is more capable than you.

We will spend the week practicing mindfulness, gratitude, and acceptance to experience the joy and peace available to us right now!

Gratitude is a sure way to reduce stress, and it will be your biggest punch against one of the more destructive hormones, cortisol. But we will dive into that in a later chapter.

I want you to know that even though you will not always know the answer, as you keep moving forward, you will find it in the future where you need it. Don't spend today worrying about tomorrow when you could be soaking in the sun.

Day one

Think about the past week and identify three strong emotions you felt. Write them down.

_____

_____

_____

_____

For each emotion, describe a specific situation that triggered it. What were you doing? Who was involved?

_____

_____

_____

_____

_____

How did these emotions affect your behavior or decision-making in those moments?

_____

_____

_____

_____

_____

_____

_____

_____

MOOD (FEEL)

☺ ☺ ☺ ☹ ☹ ☹ ☺

SAY: 10 things you are grateful for

Day two

Choose one of the emotions you wrote about on Day 1. What are the deeper triggers behind this emotion? Consider past experiences, underlying fears, or unmet needs that might be contributing.

_____

_____

_____

_____

_____

_____

From that same situation, please think of how you could reframe it to see the other side of the coin. How else could you have reacted in that instance?

_____

_____

_____

_____

_____

_____

_____

Think of the most positive person you know. How may they have handled that same situation?

_____

_____

_____

_____   MOOD (FEEL)

_____   ☺ 🙂 😐 😕 ☹ 😣 😖

Day three

Reflect on a recent time when you were hard on yourself. What were your thoughts and feelings? How would you respond to a friend in the same circumstance?

_____
_____
_____
_____
_____
_____
_____
_____
_____
_____
_____
_____
_____
_____
_____
_____
_____

Think of a time when you chose a positive reaction when it would have been easier not to do so.

_____
_____
_____
_____

MOOD (FEEL)

_____

Day Four

Reflect on how empathy could change your view on the most challenging relationship in your life. How does understanding the other person's emotions and perspective alter your feelings about the situation? (this does not include abuse; please do not try to understand an abuser)

_____
_____
_____
_____
_____
_____
_____
_____

Identify someone in your life who might be going through a tough time. What compassionate action can you take to support them?

_____
_____
_____
_____
_____

How does compassion towards others affect your emotions?

_____

MOOD (FEEL)

☺ ☺ ☺ ☺ ☺ ☺ ☺

_____
_____

Day Five

Reflect on your most challenging life experiences and list 3 of the hardest ones below

_____

_____

_____

_____

_____

_____

_____

_____

_____

_____

For each of those three, write down ONE thing you can be grateful for in each circumstance.

_____

_____

_____

_____

_____

_____

_____

_____

_____

MOOD (FEEL)

😊 😌 😐 😠 😢 😬 😶

Day Six

Reflect on moments when trusting in God brought you peace. Write about a specific time when your faith helped you overcome anxiety or worry.

_____

_____

_____

_____

_____

_____

_____

_____

Think of a current challenge you're facing. How can placing this situation in God's hands change your perspective or emotional response?

_____

_____

_____

_____

_____

_____

_____

_____

MOOD (FEEL)

😊 😌 😐 ☹️ 😣 😵 😕

Think about what it means for you to trust in God's plan, especially in times of difficulty.

_____

Day Seven

List 10 people you are thankful for and a short reason why.

_____

_____

_____

_____

_____

_____

_____

_____

_____

_____

_____

_____

_____

_____

_____

_____

_____

_____

_____

_____

MOOD (FEEL)

😊 😟 😮 😠 😢 😎 😐

Step two
Mental
Ascension

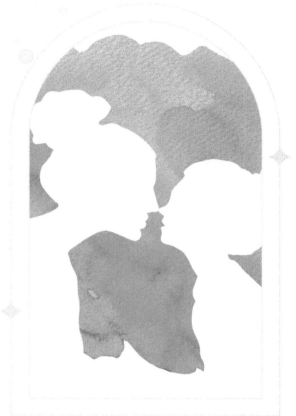

In motherhood, the most ordinary days are tinted with the extraordinary, painting love in the details of the mundane.

Becoming The Master

Now that we have talked about your mind, the center of your beliefs and thought patterns, I want us to look into the role our hormones play in how we feel daily and what exactly hormones do so that we can see the power we have to master the internal workings of our bodies. This chapter may feel very heady, so don't worry if you need help understanding it. If you are in the course, there will be a lecture shared on this topic.

If you have any hormonal imbalance, you have likely been in the back seat of your journey. It's time for you to see the power you have when you have a say in what happens inside your body.

Hormones are powerful chemical messengers produced by hubs called the endocrine glands. These glands release hormones directly into your blood, which then delivers them to the organs and tissues in your body so that they can do their work, such as regulating and controlling growth, metabolism, mood, and reproductive functions.

Think of your body as a symphony orchestra, with hormones as the musicians. Each one, from thyroid hormones to insulin, plays a specific and crucial role, and when in harmony, they create a beautiful melody and feelings of wellness; when out of balance, they sound more like chaos, which represents over 50 known symptoms of hormonal imbalance. Our goal is to understand these players and gently guide them back to their perfect pitch. Our modern lifestyles, often disconnected from nature's rhythm and wholeness, can contribute to these imbalances.

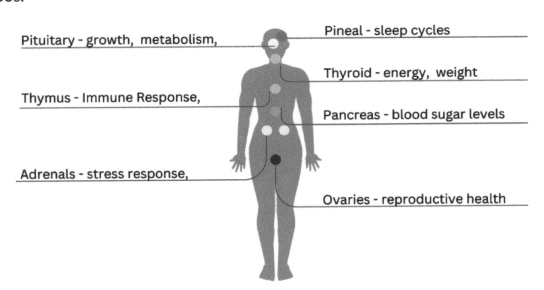

Pituitary - growth, metabolism,

Pineal - sleep cycles

Thyroid - energy, weight

Thymus - Immune Response,

Pancreas - blood sugar levels

Adrenals - stress response,

Ovaries - reproductive health

(visual summary of some of the glands and the hormones they produce)

WEEK 2

Hormonal imbalance occurs when there is too much or too little hormone in the bloodstream. Because of their importance, even slight hormonal imbalances can cause side effects throughout the body.

Below are some of the common symptoms of hormonal imbalance:

- **Fatigue**: Often one of the most common signs, a persistent feeling of tiredness can be a signal from the body that thyroid hormones, responsible for energy regulation, are out of balance.

- **Weight Gain or Loss**: Unexplained weight changes can be linked to imbalances in thyroid hormones, cortisol, insulin, and sex hormones. Each plays a distinct role in metabolism and fat storage.

- **Mood Swings and Mental Health Issues**: Hormones are deeply intertwined with brain chemistry, influencing mood and emotional well-being. Fluctuations in estrogen and progesterone, for example, can contribute to mood swings and anxiety, especially notable in conditions like Premenstrual Syndrome (PMS) or menopause.

- **Menstrual Irregularities**: In women, irregularities in the menstrual cycle, such as missed periods, heavy bleeding, or painful periods, can be indicative of hormonal imbalances, particularly involving estrogen and progesterone.

- **Sleep Disturbances**: Hormones like cortisol and melatonin play a role in sleep patterns. An imbalance can lead to insomnia or sleep disturbances.

- **Changes in Physical Appearance**: Acne, hair loss, or skin changes can often signify hormonal shifts. Androgens, a group of hormones that include testosterone, can influence the skin and hair.

Because of genetics and environmental differences, none of us are exactly alike, so we don't all have the same symptoms of hormonal imbalance. It would really help if you recognized the things that are happening in your life that may be linked to hormonal imbalances. I also encourage you to visit your primary care physician and get a test to determine exactly which hormones are out of balance, so that you have a clear picture of what you may need to do to get back in harmony.

Remember, every symptom has a cause. You may not know it, but it is worth finding out. As the CEO of your body, you determine the level of wellness you will pursue from this point forward.

Day one

If you have not done so already, please go to www.everydaynurse and look for the hormone symptom checklist, and fill it out. Remember, this is not a diagnosis but just an informational tool.

_____

_____

Have you talked to your healthcare provider about your symptoms? If, yes, how did it go? If, Not why not?

_____

_____

_____

_____

_____

_____

Describe your typical PMS days

_____

_____

_____

_____

WATER (CUPS)

◊ ◊ ◊ ◊ ◊ ◊ ◊ ◊ ◊

SLEEP (HRS)

○ ○ ○ ○ ○ ○ ○ ○ ○

MOOD (FEEL)

☺ ☺ ☺ ☹ ☹ ☺ ☺

EXERCISE (MIN)

FOOD LOG

Have you felt supported in your journey or isolated and misunderstood? Reflect on your journey and either express gratitude or forgiveness to those around you.

Day two

Do you track your cycle? Consider using an app or physical calendar to see where you are in the cycle so you can be more self-aware about your interactions. There just may be things you will have to avoid on certain days.

Think back to when you reacted to a situation and later felt like you had overreacted. Write about it in detail.

_____
_____
_____
_____
_____
_____
_____
_____
_____

Do you currently use birth control pills, patches, shots or any other chemical forms of it? have you noticed any changes in yourself since starting.

_____

_____   WATER (CUPS)
                                      ◊ ◊ ◊ ◊ ◊ ◊ ◊ ◊
_____
                                      SLEEP (HRS)
_____   ○ ○ ○ ○ ○ ○ ○ ○

_____   MOOD (FEEL)
                                      ☺ ☺ ☺ ☹ ☹ ☺ ☺
_____
                                      EXERCISE (MIN) [____]
_____
                                      FOOD LOG
_____

Day three

What is something about hormones you did not know?

_____

_____

_____

_____

_____

_____

_____

How does it change your perspective on the symptoms you have been experiencing? Do you feel a sense of hope for your future?

_____

_____

_____

_____

_____

_____

Reflect on the the last 5 years. What are 3 ways in which you have become a better person?

_____

_____

_____

_____

_____

_____

WATER (CUPS)

◊ ◊ ◊ ◊ ◊ ◊ ◊ ◊

SLEEP (HRS)

○ ○ ○ ○ ○ ○ ○ ○

MOOD (FEEL)

☺ ☻ ☺ ☹ ☹ ☺ ☺

EXERCISE (MIN)

FOOD LOG

Day Four

What are three positive things about my health or body I experienced today? How did these moments make me feel?"

_____

_____

_____

_____

_____

_____

_____

What specific aspects of my body's functionality am I grateful for today? (e.g., the ability to walk, see, hear, etc.) Come up with 10.

_____

_____

_____

_____

_____

_____

WATER (CUPS)

◊ ◊ ◊ ◊ ◊ ◊ ◊ ◊

SLEEP (HRS)

○ ○ ○ ○ ○ ○ ○ ○ ○

MOOD (FEEL)

☺ ☺ ☺ ☹ ☹ ☺ ☺

EXERCISE (MIN)

FOOD LOG

Day five

Reflect on a health challenge I faced and overcame. What strengths did my body and mind show during this time?

_____

_____

_____

_____

_____

_____

Think of the health challenges or hormonal imbalance issues you are currently facing. How can you use your strengths to overcome those challenges this time?

_____

_____

_____

_____

_____

Consider 5 things you're thankful for learning.

_____

_____

_____

_____

_____

_____

WATER (CUPS)

◊ ◊ ◊ ◊ ◊ ◊ ◊ ◊

SLEEP (HRS)

○ ○ ○ ○ ○ ○ ○ ○

MOOD (FEEL)

☺ ☺ ☺ ☹ ☹ ☺ ☺

EXERCISE (MIN)

FOOD LOG

Day Six

Interview one of the women in the program about her hormone journey and find ways to her. (If you are doing this as a self-study participant, interview a friend or family member.) The Questions could revolve around personal experiences, coping strategies, and insights gained. Reflecting on these stories can provide comfort, new perspectives, and a sense of community.

_____

_____

How did it feel to talk to someone else about their journey?

_____

_____

_____

_____

_____

_____

_____

_____

_____

_____

How important do you think it is for teen and tween girls to be educated about their hormones and how to maintain balance?

_____

_____

_____

_____

_____

_____

_____

_____

WATER (CUPS)

◊ ◊ ◊ ◊ ◊ ◊ ◊ ◊

SLEEP (HRS)

○ ○ ○ ○ ○ ○ ○ ○ ○

MOOD (FEEL)

☺ ☺ ☺ ☹ ☹ ☺ ☺

EXERCISE (MIN)

FOOD LOG

Day Seven

Gratitude Jar: Create a jar, box, or even Ziplock bag in which you write a note of gratitude about your health or body each day and drop it in. Review these notes at the end of the month.

Write a letter to yourself expressing gratitude for your health and body, acknowledging your journey and resilience.

_____

_____

_____

_____

_____

_____

_____

_____

_____

_____

_____

_____

_____

_____

_____

_____ WATER (CUPS)

_____ ⬦ ⬦ ⬦ ⬦ ⬦ ⬦ ⬦ ⬦

_____ SLEEP (HRS)

_____ ○ ○ ○ ○ ○ ○ ○ ○ ○

_____ MOOD (FEEL)

_____ ☺ ☺ ☺ ☹ ☹ ☺ ☺

_____ EXERCISE (MIN) [____]

_____ FOOD LOG

_____

_____

_____

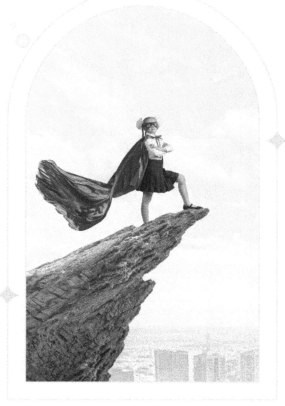

When a mother is her best self, she becomes the mirror in which her children see the brightest possibilities of their own being."

WEEK 4
The Sound of Wellness

Recently, my children and I watched a classical music masterpiece on YouTube: The Handel Messiah. A large choir performed with hundreds of people, resulting in a great listening experience thanks to a very talented Orchestra. It was incredible to watch how every musician had mastery over their instrument and knew when to chime in to make the music complete. The focus was often on the vocalists, but we know they wouldn't have sounded great without the other musicians faithfully doing their part.

In the same way, you are the vocalist in your life and the star of the show. However, some aspects of your life give you the backing and the music as you belt out your beautiful tune. These are your lifestyle habits. When your lifestyle habits are optimal, the music complements your performance. But When you decide to sustain unhealthy habits, you may belt out the finest song, but the supporting orchestra will make it all sound awful. Keep in mind that your body is interconnected, so everything affects...well, everything else.

There are eight categories that generally affect your lifestyle: mindset, sunshine, oxygen, hydration, sleep, self-regulation, diet, and exercise. We already talked about mindset in the first two weeks of this program, and I encourage you to go back to it whenever you feel like you are going backward in progress. It happens.

Most of your wellness changes can be traced to one of these. In this chapter, we will discuss self-regulation at length and then briefly touch on the other seven, which will be featured in the following chapters.

Self-regulation, also known as self-control or temperance, is the key to ensuring that your orchestra makes good music. We must select the players well and seek to surround ourselves with the best backdrop for our lives. Well, how does this work outside of this musical example (that I may have stretched too far *tee-hee*...). Self-regulation says, "Don't eat rat poison," but it also says, "Don't eat a whole bag of family-size chips in one sitting." It is about regulating our choices and being aware of our surroundings and their impact on our bodies.

We tend to be more keenly aware of the effects of some of the negative habits we sometimes allow into our lives, like smoking, alcohol, or excessive sugar consumption. Yet, we sometimes neglect to pay attention to the environmental influences causing issues in our bodies. Chemicals in household cleaners, plastics, and personal care products often contain endocrine disruptors like phthalates and BPA. These disruptors mimic our hormones, often leading to imbalances. (P.S. If you are wondering where to start, I have created a

WEEK 4

downloadable PDF with a few of the daily environmental toxins we come across and sug-gestions for more natural alternatives.)

We cannot get rid of every harmful element around us (and this should not be the goal oth-erwise you will 10X your current stress levels), but we can do our best to reduce our expo-sure. Simple changes include choosing natural, organic products, being mindful of the air quality in our homes, or the simple act of opting for alternatives to plastic.

We also have to be mindful of the environmental effects on our minds through the things we choose to see or listen to and even the company we have chosen to keep. research says that You are the sum of the five people you spend most of your time with, and that includes the people on your gadgets. If you spend time with content that is full of chaos, drama and stress, it translates into a life full of chaos and crisis. This will negatively impact your physical body as well.

Holistic health recognizes that nature and nurture both shape who you are, how your body functions, and how you relate to those around you.

let's take a quick look at the other six categories, as they will addressed in other chapters in detail.

Sunshine

We often think of the sun in terms of vitamin D production on the positive end and skin cancer on the opposite spectrum, Yet the sun's rays do so much more for our bodies. Who remembers back in the day when we would place newborns in that gentle morning sun to prevent or reverse jaundice? Who else recalls the days when you would have a wound and be instructed to let it get some sunshine to help it heal and keep it from infection? The sun also supports relaxation, often helping drop a heightened blood pressure. However, the sun is crucial to hormone health; we will explore this further in the next chapter.

Air

The most essential element for sustaining life is air. Clean, fresh air can be harder to get these days with the increasing concern for indoor air pollution. OPEN YOUR WINDOWS! Yes, even in the winter, you need the fresh air. Also, intentionally spend more time outdoors in spaces where the air is clean. Take deep, restful breaths and enjoy the instant relaxation you will feel.

WEEK 4

Water

You are mostly made up of water. It's shocking to see how some societies travel a long way for clean drinking water while others poison their clean water with dyes, chemicals, carbon dioxide (to make sodas), and high amounts of sugar before declaring it fit to drink. Water is the essence of all life and the river through which all deliveries are made, from your oxygen to your hormones and nutrients.

Rest

Sleep is a sanctuary. I almost feel like I haven't had a full night of sleep in years because I had five children in nine years. Disrupted sleep patterns can lead to hormonal imbalances, weight gain, and even insulin resistance. What's worse, you know how cranky we can be when we don't get enough sleep! Long-term sleep deprivation can have significant health consequences.

Nutrition

A diet rich in essential nutrients is one of the most underrated elements of wellness. As a society, we have traveled further and further away from whole foods that provide elemental building blocks for our physical, mental, and emotional well-being. Many of us feel the effect of that lack in our hormonal imbalances. Food is the Lego pieces that make up our entire body and fuel our minds.

Most ailments begin in our mouths and can end in our mouths if we embrace food as medicine. Your body can overhaul its cells and build a new system in a few days. So, if you start feeding yourself better, you will see the positive effects very rapidly!

Exercise

Exercise is often linked to weight loss, but it is far more essential to our existence than just a tool for weight loss. Exercise is essential for heart health, muscle tone, bone strength, mental clarity, better metabolism, excellent blood flow, Detox through sweat, feel-good hormone production, oxygenation of cells, and SO MUCH MORE!

In addition, exercise is a natural antidote to stress. Exercise is one of the most underutilized preventative measures for many illnesses.

Day one

Fill out the Lifestyle Assessment download available on www.EverydayNurse.com/tools and write down the areas of your life that you would like to work on

_____

_____

_____

_____

_____

_____

_____

What is your weakest category? How did it get that way?

_____

_____

_____

_____

_____

WATER (CUPS)

◇ ◇ ◇ ◇ ◇ ◇ ◇ ◇

_____

SLEEP (HRS)

○ ○ ○ ○ ○ ○ ○ ○

_____

MOOD (FEEL)

☺ ☺ ☺ ☹ ☹ ☺ ☹

EXERCISE (MIN) [   ]

_____

FOOD LOG

Think of your current daily routine and schedule; how can you make room for some new habits? Remember, easy does it. Some habits need just 30 seconds a day to start with.

Day two

Make a list of 5 things you're doing right in your lifestyle choices.

_____
_____
_____
_____
_____
_____
_____
_____

Do you feel like you are too hard on yourself when you miss the mark on the goals you set? If so, can you write a paragraph encouraging yourself.

_____
_____
_____
_____

WATER (CUPS)

◊ ◊ ◊ ◊ ◊ ◊ ◊ ◊

SLEEP (HRS)

◯ ◯ ◯ ◯ ◯ ◯ ◯ ◯

MOOD (FEEL)

☺ ☺ ☺ ☹ ☹ ☺ ☺

EXERCISE (MIN) [   ]

FOOD LOG

Day three

What do you feel is in your home environment that causes stress to you mentally or contributes to your hormone imbalance?

_____

_____

_____

_____

_____

_____

_____

Research and write down one thing you are committed to change in order to reduce the mental or physical stress

_____

_____

_____

_____

_____

_____

How do you feel about losing specific patterns, habits, and products?

_____

_____

_____

_____

_____

WATER (CUPS)

○ ○ ○ ○ ○ ○ ○ ○

SLEEP (HRS)

○ ○ ○ ○ ○ ○ ○ ○

MOOD (FEEL)

☺ ☺ ☺ ☹ ☹ ☺ ☹

EXERCISE (MIN)

FOOD LOG

Day Four

How are you feeling today? (vent session)

_____

_____

_____

_____

_____

_____

_____

Read your vent and try to find the underlying feeling behind any negative expressions you wrote. Use the tools from week one and two to reframe your thoughts.

_____

_____

_____

_____

_____

_____

Write 5 things you like most about yourself TODAY!

_____

_____

_____

_____

_____

_____

WATER (CUPS)

◊ ◊ ◊ ◊ ◊ ◊ ◊ ◊

SLEEP (HRS)

○ ○ ○ ○ ○ ○ ○ ○

MOOD (FEEL)

☺ ☺ ☺ ☹ ☹ ☺ ☹

EXERCISE (MIN)

FOOD LOG

Day five

Why are you going through this program? What does this transformation mean to you. Dig deep and remind yourself of your why

_____

_____

_____

_____

_____

_____

List 10 things you would like to get rid of in your life. (You may list food items, physical products that may be interfering with your progress, habits that you may want to break, toxic cleaning products, stuff that is causing clutter and keeping your mind in chaos, etc.) In the next column, List 10 things you would like to implement as a replacement.

_____	_____
_____	_____
_____	_____
_____	_____

WATER (CUPS)

○ ○ ○ ○ ○ ○ ○ ○

SLEEP (HRS)

○ ○ ○ ○ ○ ○ ○ ○

MOOD (FEEL)

☺ ☺ ☺ ☹ ☹ ☺ ☺

EXERCISE (MIN)

FOOD LOG

Day Six

You are becoming someone more familiar to yourself, but this person may be new to those around you. What are you most excited about having your loved ones learn about you?

_____

_____

_____

_____

_____

_____

As you look back at who you used to be when you felt most alive, beautiful, and happy, Think of some of the elements from that version of self that you no longer want to bring into this more mature, radiant you.

_____

_____

_____

_____

_____

_____

_____

_____

_____

_____

WATER (CUPS)

○ ○ ○ ○ ○ ○ ○ ○

SLEEP (HRS)

○ ○ ○ ○ ○ ○ ○ ○

MOOD (FEEL)

☺ ☺ ☺ ☹ ☹ ☺ ☺

EXERCISE (MIN)

FOOD LOG

Day Seven

Write a letter to a loved one of your choice. Empty yourself of gratitude for them, and find positive aspects of them you have never seen before. Some may be hiding behind things that may be seen as annoyances. You do not have to show it to them if you choose. This is an exercise to benefit you more than them

_____

_____

_____

_____

_____

_____

_____

_____

_____

_____

_____

_____

_____

_____

_____

_____   **WATER (CUPS)**

_____   ◊ ◊ ◊ ◊ ◊ ◊ ◊ ◊

_____   **SLEEP (HRS)**

_____   ○ ○ ○ ○ ○ ○ ○ ○ ○

_____   **MOOD (FEEL)**

_____   ☺ ☺ ☺ ☹ ☹ ☺ ☹

_____   **EXERCISE (MIN)**

_____   **FOOD LOG**

_____

Step three

Physical Activation

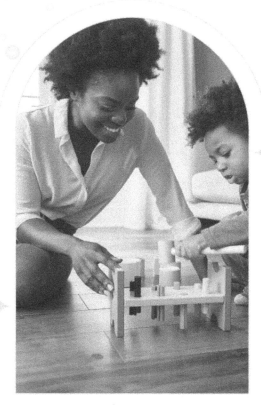

Through the simple act of play, a mother lays the foundation of love, joy, and trust, crafting memories that build the bridge between hearts and shaping the future with laughter and connection.

WEEK 5

Inhale Your Vibrant Future

Have you thought it interesting that after God created Adam, He physically breathed into his nostrils? God did not have to do that; He could have spoken or thought it. But the breath was so vital that God Himself delivered the first Life awakening breath into Adam. The beauty of life is that each day, we still receive breath as a gift, and it is our responsibility to enjoy each inhalation and make it as fresh and full of life and vigor as possible. Step outside of yesterday, out of all the failures, out of the pain, the disappointments that keep you stuck there, and move into today, take the present breath. Breathe.

Oxygen is the most critical element for the continuation of life, and we must be intentional about getting clean air around us. Have you ever noticed how fresh air can instantly clear your mind and sharpen your focus? This is because oxygen helps improve concentration and mental clarity. Deep breathing also calms your mind, helping to ease the stress, tension, and anxiety that are often linked with hormone imbalance. So whenever you're feeling over-whelmed, try to go outside and take some deep breaths, you will feel better almost instant-ly. Remember, your body is like a circle, so if your cells are well-oxygenated and working well, your whole body benefits from it.

As a mother, it's crucial to prioritize self-care, and spending time outdoors, even with your little ones, can be an excellent way to nourish your body and soul while bonding with your family. Simple activities like picnicking at a park or playing tag in the backyard can be very beneficial for your sense of balance. It does not have to be planned or complicated.

A second benefit of being outdoors is being exposed to sunshine. The morning and evening sun are the best for our enjoyment (and selfies!). Sunshine is most commonly known for helping our bodies make Vitamin D, drying out wounds, and even helping newborns process jaundice, but it does so much more for us. Being in the sun can help reduce stress and even help reset our internal clock. This clock, known as the circadian rhythm, is responsible for your sleepiness and helps you stay asleep on the sun's cycle.

Vitamin D is necessary for many functions in our bodies, including hormone production.

This week, I want you to think of how much time you spend outdoors daily and begin to make small changes to be more intentional about giving your lungs deep, full breaths of air while giving your skin a gentle glow from the sun.

WEEK 5

This week marks the beginning of the physical changes you will make in your quest to find balance. Some will be easy, and some challenging, but I would like you to remember your WHY... keep it close. Write it on a piece of paper and post it on your wall. If you are in the 12-week Program online, you will be journeying with others, and we will definitely keep you accountable and surrounded by loving support that reminds you that 'YOU. CAN. DO.' THIS. Wherever you are, there is a team cheering for you; some are close to you, and others, like myself, are further away, but we believe in you!

Be prepared for the internal resistance that you will face as you change. Remember what you learned in the first two chapters. These lessons will accompany you every time you face change, and you can always go back and read them anytime you need to.

OK, please take a deep breath because talking about it can sometimes bring tension. And another deep breath... that's better. But just in case you need it, let's go a third round ... .innnnnn and blow that air ouuuuuuuuut.

Whenever I do this, I feel so much lighter, and it is often accompanied by a smile breaking on my lips as if my body fills with peace as it remembers its Creator, who breathed in the very first breath.

Day one

Go to your favorite fresh air spot and practice deep breathing. Inhale as much as you can, then take in a little more; as you let it out, think of all the stress and anxiety you want to release and let it go with the breath as you blow it out.

Write about a time when you felt like going outside to take in a few deep breaths or take a walk in order to feel better either physically or mentally

_____

_____

_____

_____

_____

Think of one of your favorite childhood memories of being outside and write it down in detail. (if you don't have any, think of a video, book, or any positive memory from your past)

_____

_____

_____

_____

_____

_____

_____

WATER (CUPS)

◊ ◊ ◊ ◊ ◊ ◊ ◊ ◊

SLEEP (HRS)

○ ○ ○ ○ ○ ○ ○ ○

MOOD (FEEL)

☺ ☺ ☺ ☹ ☹ ☺ ☺

EXERCISE (MIN)

FOOD LOG

Day two

Step outside. Go for a 10-minute walk or activity.

How was your time outside? What did you do or see? How did it feel? Try to recall as much detail as possible and write it all down.

_____

_____

_____

_____

_____

_____

_____

_____

_____

_____

_____

_____

_____

Do you feel like an outdoors or indoors person? What is the source of that feeling?

_____

_____

_____

_____

_____

_____

WATER (CUPS)

◊ ◊ ◊ ◊ ◊ ◊ ◊ ◊ ◊

SLEEP (HRS)

○ ○ ○ ○ ○ ○ ○ ○ ○

MOOD (FEEL)

☺ ☺ ☺ ☺ ☺ ☺ ☺

EXERCISE (MIN)

FOOD LOG

Day Three

What are five things you enjoy doing outside?

_____

_____

_____

_____

_____

_____

_____

_____

Out of those five activities, think of two you did within the last month and write down what the experience was like for you.

_____

_____

_____

_____

_____

_____

_____

Think of some of your daily activities you could do while outdoors (e.g, opening the mail and organizing bills)

_____

_____

_____

_____

_____

WATER (CUPS)

⬦ ⬦ ⬦ ⬦ ⬦ ⬦ ⬦ ⬦

SLEEP (HRS)

◯ ◯ ◯ ◯ ◯ ◯ ◯ ◯

MOOD (FEEL)

☺ ☹ ☺ ☹ ☹ ☺ ☹

EXERCISE (MIN)

FOOD LOG

Day Four

Please research ten health benefits of spending time in the sun. Write your findings below.

_____

_____

_____

_____

_____

_____

_____

_____

_____

_____

_____

_____

_____

_____

How did this exercise change how you view spending time in the sun?

_____

_____

_____

_____

_____

_____

WATER (CUPS)

○ ○ ○ ○ ○ ○ ○ ○

SLEEP (HRS)

○ ○ ○ ○ ○ ○ ○ ○

MOOD (FEEL)

☺ ☺ ☺ ☹ ☹ ☺ ☺

EXERCISE (MIN)

FOOD LOG

Day five

What keeps you from spending more time outside

_____
_____
_____
_____
_____
_____
_____

Share 3 positive emotions you feel when you are outside.

_____
_____
_____
_____
_____
_____
_____

Which of the positive emotions you listed above is
most valuable to you and why?

WATER (CUPS)

⬯ ⬯ ⬯ ⬯ ⬯ ⬯ ⬯ ⬯

SLEEP (HRS)

○ ○ ○ ○ ○ ○ ○ ○ ○ ○

MOOD (FEEL)

☺ 😐 🙂 😖 😢 😀 😑

EXERCISE (MIN) ☐

FOOD LOG

Day Six

Make a plan to take your family on an outdoor activity next week. Write down in detail how great it will be, imagine the joy and laughter, and paint a word picture to create a joyful anticipation for this activity next week

_____

_____

_____

_____

_____

_____

_____

_____

_____

_____

_____

_____

List 5 things you are thankful for

_____

_____

_____

_____

_____

WATER (CUPS)

SLEEP (HRS)

MOOD (FEEL)

EXERCISE (MIN)

FOOD LOG

Day Seven

Write a poem about the sights and sounds, creatures and/or experiences you have encountered outdoors.

_____

_____

_____

_____

_____

_____

_____

_____

_____

_____

_____

_____

WATER (CUPS)

◊ ◊ ◊ ◊ ◊ ◊ ◊ ◊

SLEEP (HRS)

○ ○ ○ ○ ○ ○ ○ ○

MOOD (FEEL)

☺ ☺ ☺ ☹ ☹ ☺ ☹

EXERCISE (MIN)

FOOD LOG

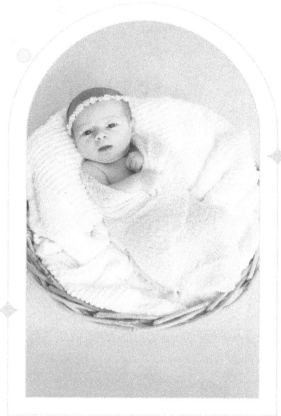

"The art of mothering is
to teach the art
of living to children."

– Elaine Heffner

Hydrate to Elevate

Oh dear! I have to tell on myself... Some days, I wake up and pee before I start my morning routine, and then I find myself only returning to the bathroom to pee again in the evening. It's easy for me to forget to hydrate unless I am intentional about it. That a hard truth to admit right before I write about the AMAZING benefits of drinking water. Water accounts for about 70% of our body structure, and we need to keep this water machine watered! That was a lot.

When I fall behind on my water intake and get dehydrated it is tough to get hydrated again. It seems like when those days happen and I start drinking water, the water just runs out of me and I remain feeling like a prune. My lips will be dry, my mind will be sluggish and my skin loses its supple glow. It's just not worth it!

Your body NEEDS water, constantly. As you go through your day, you continually lose water through your skin, breathing, bathroom trips, and whenever you open your mouth to chat. Maintaining proper hydration is about replacing the water we constantly lose in our body by drinking the recommended amounts of water for our age, activity levels, and body weight. The standard 6-8 cups of water is a great place to start, but you should aim to personalize that number as it changes based on your lifestyle and needs. For example, a breastfeeding mother needs more water because she uses much of it to make milk for her little one.

Because the brain is made up of close to 90% water, the sensibility of your thoughts, feelings, and decisions greatly depends on us keeping the brain well hydrated. Water is not merely a thirst quencher; it's a critical component of our day-to-day lives.

Some people don't like the taste of water, which is understandable. Remember, you like what you eat and eat what you want, which also goes for drinks. Your taste buds become adapted to whatever they are given. To begin with, you could add some lemon or mint leaves to your water so that it gets a flavor of sorts and doesn't taste as plain. For some, you may have to start by diluting parts of the beverages you are used to and adding bits of water until it's mostly water, and then you can stop adding the beverage. It may take days or weeks, but it's worth the journey.

Internally, proper hydration helps maintain our blood flow, which helps transport hormones throughout the body. Below are some ways in which hydration is linked to balance.

WEEK 6

Stress Management: Water plays a vital role in regulating the levels of stress hormones like cortisol. When you're dehydrated, your body may produce more cortisol, making you feel more stressed and anxious.

Balance and Energy Levels: Proper hydration is essential for maintaining stable energy levels and a positive mood. Dehydration can lead to changes in hormone levels that control energy and mood, leaving you feeling tired, irritable, or even down.

Metabolism: Water is involved in many metabolic processes, including those related to thyroid hormones that regulate metabolism. When dehydrated, thyroid function can be affected, potentially slowing metabolism and making it harder to manage weight.

Reproductive Health: Hydration is essential for reproductive hormone balance in both men and women. Dehydration can disrupt hormone levels involved in fertility and reproductive health. Staying hydrated may support the proper functioning of hormones like estrogen and testosterone, which are essential for reproductive health.

As you can see, drinking enough water isn't just that thing we were constantly reminded to do as children (thanks, Mom!); it's an absolute necessity to keep this water structure, our body, working at its best. This week, we will begin practicing good water habits together. I have a tool you can download from the website www.EverydayNurse.com, and it has suggestions on how you can incorporate more water into your daily life based on things I have done for me and my family to drink more water.

Day one

Reflect on your current hydration habits. How many glasses of water do you drink daily? Are there specific times or seasons when you find it hard to stay hydrated? What can you do to improve it

_____

_____

_____

_____

_____

_____

_____

Use the online calculators to find out how much water you should drink based on your weight, activity levels, and lifestyle. Write that number down and then make a plan on how you can slowly get to that number

_____

_____

_____

_____

_____

_____

_____

_____

_____

WATER (CUPS)

◊ ◊ ◊ ◊ ◊ ◊ ◊ ◊ ◊

SLEEP (HRS)

○ ○ ○ ○ ○ ○ ○ ○ ○

MOOD (FEEL)

☺ ☺ ☺ ☹ ☹ ☺ ☺

EXERCISE (MIN)

FOOD LOG

Carry a water bottle with you all day. Track your drinking habits and how they your mood and energy levels.

Day two

Take time to think of your barriers to drinking water and write them all down.

_____

_____

_____

_____

_____

_____

_____

What do you drink daily besides water? How does it add to or take away from your hydration goals? Do some research if needed.

_____

_____

_____

_____

_____

WATER (CUPS)

○ ○ ○ ○ ○ ○ ○ ○ ○

SLEEP (HRS)

○ ○ ○ ○ ○ ○ ○ ○ ○

MOOD (FEEL)

☺ ☺ ☺ ☹ ☹ ☺ ☺

EXERCISE (MIN)

FOOD LOG

Day Three

Consider your body's signals of dehydration. What signs do you typically experience first? How can you better tune in to these signals?

_____

_____

_____

_____

_____

_____

_____

Think of 7 positive words or feelings that you can associate with drinking water.

_____

_____

_____

_____

_____

_____

_____

_____

_____

_____

_____

WATER (CUPS)

SLEEP (HRS)

MOOD (FEEL)

EXERCISE (MIN)

FOOD LOG

Day Four

What have you put in place to help you drink more water? How are those cues working for you?

_____

_____

_____

_____

_____

_____

Incorporate a glass of water about 15-20 min before each meal. Notice if it affects your hunger levels, how you enjoy your food, or your portion sizes.

_____

_____

_____

_____

_____

WATER (CUPS)

◊ ◊ ◊ ◊ ◊ ◊ ◊ ◊

SLEEP (HRS)

○ ○ ○ ○ ○ ○ ○ ○

MOOD (FEEL)

☺ ☹ ☺ ☹ ☹ ☺ ☺

EXERCISE (MIN)

FOOD LOG

Research: How hydration affects your hormonal balance and symptoms.

Day five

Do you drink more water when you are out or at home? Why do you think that is?

_____

_____

_____

_____

_____

_____

Look up, signs of dehydration and list all that have affected you at some point.

_____

_____

_____

_____

_____

_____

_____

WATER (CUPS)

○ ○ ○ ○ ○ ○ ○ ○ ○

SLEEP (HRS)

○ ○ ○ ○ ○ ○ ○ ○ ○

MOOD (FEEL)

☺ ☺ ☺ ☹ ☹ ☺ ☺

EXERCISE (MIN) [   ]

FOOD LOG

[   ]

Set reminders on your phone, place water bottles in key locations (work desk, living area), or pair drinking water with specific daily tasks or habits.

Day Six

What sustainable changes can you make to your daily routine to help you maintain stay hydrated

_____

_____

_____

_____

_____

_____

_____

What structures have you established to help you continue in the right direction?

_____

_____

_____

_____

_____

_____

_____

List 5 things you are thankful for

_____

_____

_____

_____

_____

WATER (CUPS)

◊ ◊ ◊ ◊ ◊ ◊ ◊ ◊

SLEEP (HRS)

○ ○ ○ ○ ○ ○ ○ ○

MOOD (FEEL)

☺ ☺ ☺ ☺ ☹ ☺ ☺

EXERCISE (MIN)

FOOD LOG

Day Seven

Write an encouraging letter to yourself highlighting the importance of hydration in your life based on what you've learned and experienced this week. Seal it and set a reminder to open it in one month as a check-in with yourself.

_____

_____

_____

_____

_____

_____

_____

_____

_____

_____

_____

_____

_____

_____

_____

_____

WATER (CUPS)

◇ ◇ ◇ ◇ ◇ ◇ ◇ ◇

SLEEP (HRS)

○ ○ ○ ○ ○ ○ ○ ○

MOOD (FEEL)

☺ ☺ ☺ ☹ ☹ ☺ ☺

EXERCISE (MIN)

FOOD LOG

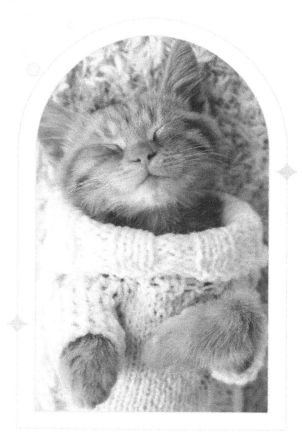

A mother's rest is as
essential as her love,
for in her calm, the
family finds its
rhythm.

Dreams of Balance

What is the deal with children resisting sleep?! Around the time they become toddlers, they become sleep-resistant ninjas! They cry before naps and cry about going to bed, only to be fast asleep 5 minutes later. Then there are the dreaded bedtime routines featuring tired parents and cranky little ones. In fact, I am ashamed to say, but some of my least shiny parenting moments have been featured at bedtime. What's funny is, In a few years, they will be adults, longing for a nap without much time or opportunity to do so.

Sleep is the thing we love to hate as children but hate to love as adults. I'm sleepy just thinking about it... yawwwn. But seriously, let's talk more about sleep, what it does for our bodies, how much we need, and how we can get more.

Sleep renews and refreshes our system and is so vital to the human body that a lack of it can make us go crazy, like actual psychosis. There is a study that found that being awake for very long periods can be similar to being under the influence of alcohol. Your body needs sleep to function well physically and mentally. When it comes to our balance, Numerous hormones, including cortisol, insulin, and the growth and hunger hormones, are regulated and aided by processes that happen in the early parts of the night due to the moon cycles and circadian rhythm (our internal clock that mirrors the sun's cycle). A lack of quality sleep can disrupt these hormones, leading to various health issues. I have summarized the science of sleep and hormones below so you can see how different stages of sleep affect your hormones and what happens when your sleep cycle is disrupted.

Fall asleep faster: Melatonin, often referred to as the "sleep hormone," helps regulate the sleep-wake cycle, promoting feelings of drowsiness and preparing the body for restorative sleep. Going to bed earlier allows your body to produce melatonin, helping you fall asleep faster and experience more restful sleep.

Feel more rested: During deep sleep stages, particularly in the first half of the night, the body releases higher levels of growth hormone (GH). Growth hormones play a crucial role in the body's repair and development. Going to bed earlier helps your body release enough of this hormone.

Think better: Sleep is essential for your brain function. Research suggests that the brain processes and organizes memories during the first half of the night. Going to bed earlier allows for more time spent in these critical stages of sleep, enhancing memory retention, learning, and cognitive performance. (The hours before midnight are worth double the hours after midnight!)

Boost immunity: Sleep plays a vital role in immune function, helping the body defend against infections and illness. According to Research, specific immune cells are more active during sleep, and sleep deprivation can negatively affect immune function. When you go to bed earlier, you allow your immune system to strengthen and recharge, which improves your wellness.

Reduce stress: Adequate sleep during the early part of the night is essential for regulating stress hormones such as cortisol. Cortisol levels typically decline during sleep, with the lowest levels occurring in the late evening and early part of the night.

Okay, so I hope you caught my not-so-subtle repetitive statement about going to sleep earlier. It is incredibly crucial that we sleep earlier, even just for beauty reasons. Do you know that you may look more youthful if you get more sleep? I hope thats all the convincing you need.

What is enough sleep, though? This varies for different people, but you want to get an average of 6-8 hours of peaceful sleep a night. There are seasons when you may not achieve this (like when you have a newborn or a sick child), and it is okay. Just try to rest whenever you can during the day and reduce your optional stressors.

This week, we will work on sleep hygiene practices, and I'd like to challenge you to assess your sleep habits and work towards eliminating the things that are costing you sleep and throwing off your hormones, leading to even more sleeplessness.

Please be sure to check out EverydayNurse.com/tools. There is a sleep hygiene tool full of best sleep practices and suggestions, and you could find this very useful for your sleep journey.

Day one

Describe your sleep environment in great detail, the feel, the colors, the sounds

_____

_____

_____

_____

_____

_____

_____

_____

_____

_____

Make a list of five small changes you can make to improve the space you sleep in.

_____

_____

_____

WATER (CUPS)

◊ ◊ ◊ ◊ ◊ ◊ ◊ ◊

_____

SLEEP (HRS)

◯ ◯ ◯ ◯ ◯ ◯ ◯ ◯

_____

MOOD (FEEL)

☺ ☺ ☺ ☺ ☹ ☺ ☺

EXERCISE (MIN) [   ]

_____

FOOD LOG

Look at the list in the question above and make one
of the easiest changes today.

Day two

What time do you go to bed daily? Do you have a set routine you practice before bed? If so, write it down; if not, it's time to make one.

_____

_____

_____

_____

_____

_____

_____

_____

Share 10 relaxing activities you can do before bed that do not involve a gadget or screen.

_____

_____

_____

_____

_____

_____

WATER (CUPS)

⬭ ⬭ ⬭ ⬭ ⬭ ⬭ ⬭ ⬭

_____

SLEEP (HRS)

◯ ◯ ◯ ◯ ◯ ◯ ◯ ◯

_____

MOOD (FEEL)

☺ ☺ ☺ ☹ ☹ ☺ ☺

EXERCISE (MIN)

FOOD LOG

Select one from the list above and set the alarm to do it tonight.

Day Three

Do you currently use medications, supplements, or herbs to help you fall asleep? Please write down why (if you do) or why not (if you do not)

_____
_____
_____
_____
_____
_____
_____

Are you satisfied with your answer above? Is your choice serving you well? If not, what would you like to change?

_____
_____
_____
_____
_____
_____

WATER (CUPS)

⬭ ⬭ ⬭ ⬭ ⬭ ⬭ ⬭ ⬭

Whats your favorite sleep memory?

SLEEP (HRS)

◯ ◯ ◯ ◯ ◯ ◯ ◯ ◯

_____

MOOD (FEEL)

☺ ☻ ☺ ☹ ☹ ☺ ☺

_____

EXERCISE (MIN) [   ]

_____

FOOD LOG

_____
_____

Day Four

How do you manage stress and anxiety before bedtime?

_____

_____

_____

_____

_____

_____

_____

Do you use electronic devices within the hour before bed? Write a plan to stop the habit. An example is using a timer (from big box stores) to turn off the WIFI in your home at a certain time each night.

_____

_____

_____

_____

_____

_____

_____

_____

_____

_____

WATER (CUPS)

◊ ◊ ◊ ◊ ◊ ◊ ◊ ◊

SLEEP (HRS)

○ ○ ○ ○ ○ ○ ○ ○

MOOD (FEEL)

☺ ☺ ☺ ☹ ☹ ☺ ☺

EXERCISE (MIN) _____

Get a bedside journal, and each day before bed, Write down five things you did right that day, five things you think you did wrong and how you can do it better next time, and five things you are thankful for. This can help you offload the thoughts coming to your mind while trying to fall asleep.

FOOD LOG

_____

Day five

Describe your diet close to bedtime. Do you eat a heavy dinner? Are you a late-night snacker.... What do you snack on? Write it all down in detail, describing a typical night.

_____

_____

_____

_____

_____

_____

_____

_____

Do you eat sleep-friendly foods high in calcium, magnesium, and tryptophan? List the ones that are common in your diet. (don't worry if these seem foreign to you; hop onto the tool tab at EverydayNurse.com and find a sleep-healthy diet tool kit you use to see which foods those would be)

_____

_____

_____

_____

Think of a way to add more sleep-friendly foods into your diet.

_____

_____

_____

_____

_____

WATER (CUPS)

◊ ◊ ◊ ◊ ◊ ◊ ◊ ◊

SLEEP (HRS)

○ ○ ○ ○ ○ ○ ○ ○

MOOD (FEEL)

☺ ～ ☺ ☹ ☹ ☺ ☺

EXERCISE (MIN)

FOOD LOG

Day Six

Are harmful habits/ addictions affecting your sleep either on a physical or thought level? Make a plan on how you are going to address these habits, including excessive screen usage. (please seek professional help if you need it; it will be well worth your time and the beauty it will bring into your life)

_____

_____

_____

_____

_____

Write down what you see as an ideal sleep schedule, environment, and pattern for your life. describe all the details of how that imagination feels to you and how you see yourself in that ideal sleep environment.

_____

_____

_____

_____

_____

_____

WATER (CUPS)

○ ○ ○ ○ ○ ○ ○ ○

SLEEP (HRS)

○ ○ ○ ○ ○ ○ ○ ○

MOOD (FEEL)

☺ ☺ ☺ ☺ ☺ ☺ ☺

EXERCISE (MIN) [   ]

FOOD LOG

[   ]

Day Seven

How would you describe your faith? Write the journey in detail.

_____

_____

_____

_____

_____

_____

_____

_____

_____

_____

_____

_____

Select Spiritual practices you would like to incorporate into your sleep routine.

_____

_____

_____

_____   WATER (CUPS)

_____   ◊ ◊ ◊ ◊ ◊ ◊ ◊ ◊

_____   SLEEP (HRS)

_____   ○ ○ ○ ○ ○ ○ ○ ○

_____   MOOD (FEEL)

_____   ☺ ☹ ☺ ☹ ☹ ☺ ☹

_____   EXERCISE (MIN) [   ]

_____   FOOD LOG

_____   ┌─────────────────┐
                                                  │   │
_____   │   │
                                                  │   │
_____   └─────────────────┘

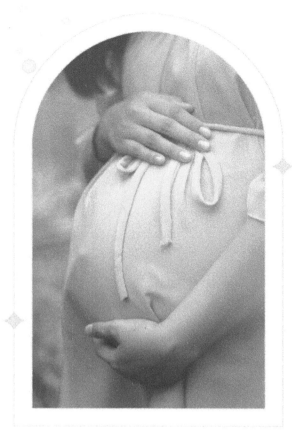

"Exercise is a celebration of what your body can do, not a punishment for what you ate."

-Anonymous

WEEK 8

Life Beyond the Scale

I sometimes feel sorry for the word exercise because weight loss stole its identity! When we hear the word exercise, there is an underlying negative feeling, instant defenses and excuses, and an internal urge to promote body positivity and self-love. Yet the point of exercise is so far from weight loss, although weight loss can sometimes be the natural side effect of exercising, even though some people exercise to bulk up and gain mass. So let's give exercise back its birthright and allow it to be the tool that helps us maintain excellent circulation, enhance our mood by producing endorphins (feel-good hormones), reduce stress and anxiety, boost our resilience, increase our energy levels by like a thousand percent!, help with pain management... ALL while also helping us achieve and or maintain a desired target weight. Okay, that was a lot, but I hope you see that exercise is NOT synonymous with weight loss.

Exercise can take on many different forms, and based on your life season, you may adapt to the form of exercise that best suits you. We often complicate the idea of exercising, which makes it feel hard and sometimes expensive and unsustainable. We need to go back and take notes from the exercise experts: little children. Have you ever seen a child at a park running, laughing, falling, getting up, and doing it again? That about sums up what we should be doing. There are no hard and fast rules; the only requirement is movement. If you have little ones around you and are unsure where to start, take them into an environment where they can be free and join them in whatever they do. You can be a play intern for the day.

You'll notice a profound thing: children have bursts of play followed by rest periods. And they cycle this over and over again. That pattern is mirrored in the now famous 'High-Intensity Interval Training' Model of exercise, which many exercise experts promote. It is super beginner-friendly because you can customize your movement time vs. your rest time and keep changing as you feel ready. I'll give you an example of how this works. About ten months After the birth of my fourth child, I started a jump rope routine where I would jump for 30 seconds, take 3-minute breaks, and do 3 to 6 cycles of that at a time. I gradually extended the 30-second jumps by ten seconds each week and reduced the break time until I started jumping for 3 minutes and taking 30-second breaks. Six cycles of this routine completed my workout for the day, and I saw drastic improvements. So remember, start slow and set yourself up for success by giving yourself some crazy-easy-no-brainer goals.

WEEK 8

Regular exercise is essential for women, especially in our productive years. Physical activity can help regulate estrogen and progesterone levels, leading to more predictable menstrual cycles and reduced symptoms of hormonal imbalances such as irregular periods, mood swings, and PMS. Regular exercise can also increase our metabolism and improve insulin sensitivity, preventing insulin resistance (which can lead to type 2 diabetes) and hormonal imbalances associated with conditions like polycystic ovary syndrome (PCOS). The benefits are not just limited to hormone health. A part of the preventative measures for conditions such as cardiovascular disease, osteoporosis, and certain cancers is adding exercise to your daily routine. Exercise, in its simplest form, is like medicine for your body.

As an added Bonus, Exercise has been shown to help you fall asleep faster and stay asleep better. Since we just completed the chapter on sleep, I hope you can see more of why it is important to take a holistic approach to your wellness. Everything is connected!

Exercise should not feel like a chore, even if initially it may feel like it. Getting started with anything is always the hardest part, and soon, your body will crave it because of all the extra energy you will have, the clarity, and the feel-good hormones that are released when you exercise. The key is finding activities you can genuinely enjoy - so try out several things and make it sustainable. The fewer barriers you remove, like going to a gym, getting exercise equipment, or getting expensive programs, the more likely you are to exercise sustainably. So, seek out routines you can do from home without tools or expense. YouTube is a great place to search for exercise channels that can inspire you and give you a sense of community by sticking with a particular content creator you like.

Nurse Tip: If you have any health challenges and need to speak to your health Care Provider before starting any activities, definitely do so.

Day one

Why is exercise essential? write down 7 reasons and research some if you have to

_____

_____

_____

_____

_____

_____

_____

_____

_____

What is your personal journey with exercise? Share the journey in detail.

_____

_____

_____

_____

_____

WATER (CUPS)

◊ ◊ ◊ ◊ ◊ ◊ ◊ ◊

SLEEP (HRS)

○ ○ ○ ○ ○ ○ ○ ○

MOOD (FEEL)

☺ ☺ ☺ ☹ ☹ ☺ ☺

EXERCISE (MIN) [   ]

FOOD LOG

[   ]

Day two

What's your ideal exercise routine? Write out your ideal scenario and place yourself in it, as if you are already doing it.

_____

_____

_____

_____

_____

_____

_____

_____

_____

_____

_____

_____

What negative thoughts come up when you think about exercising? What is the source of these thoughts

_____

_____

_____

_____

_____

_____

_____

WATER (CUPS)

◊ ◊ ◊ ◊ ◊ ◊ ◊ ◊

SLEEP (HRS)

○ ○ ○ ○ ○ ○ ○ ○

MOOD (FEEL)

☺ ☺ ☺ ☹ ☹ ☺ ☺

EXERCISE (MIN)

FOOD LOG

Day three

Step outside with a glass of water. Take 5 deep breaths, relax and then drink your water. While you drink the water, think of all the good the water is going to do in your body. Say a prayer of gratitude for clean water, outdoors and your incredible body!

Think of a time when you were consistent with exercise or play. Write about it, even if it is from childhood.

_____

_____

_____

_____

_____

_____

_____

_____

_____

Share 5 things you are you thankful for

_____

_____

_____

_____

WATER (CUPS)

○ ○ ○ ○ ○ ○ ○ ○

SLEEP (HRS)

○ ○ ○ ○ ○ ○ ○ ○ ○ ○

MOOD (FEEL)

☺ ☺ ☺ ☹ ☹ ☺ ☺

EXERCISE (MIN)

FOOD LOG

Day Four

What are the three biggest challenges that prevent you from exercising regularly?

_____

_____

_____

_____

_____

_____

_____

Brainstorm practical solutions for each barrier.

_____

_____

_____

_____

_____

_____

_____

WATER (CUPS)

◊ ◊ ◊ ◊ ◊ ◊ ◊ ◊

SLEEP (HRS)

○ ○ ○ ○ ○ ○ ○ ○

MOOD (FEEL)

☺ ☺ ☺ ☹ ☹ ☺ ☺

EXERCISE (MIN) _____

FOOD LOG

Go for a short leisurely walk. Pay attention to how your body feels with each step and your mood shifts during the walk.

Day five

How is exercise week going (vent and release)

_____
_____
_____
_____
_____
_____
_____
_____

What would make your exercise habits more successful?

_____
_____
_____
_____
_____
_____

WATER (CUPS)

◇ ◇ ◇ ◇ ◇ ◇ ◇ ◇

_____

SLEEP (HRS)

○ ○ ○ ○ ○ ○ ○ ○

_____

MOOD (FEEL)

☺ ～ ☺ ☹ ☹ ☻ ☺

_____

EXERCISE (MIN) [   ]

_____

FOOD LOG

Please join local or online support groups that will
have women with like-minded pursuits.

Day Six

Body positivity is a great thing; appreciate the body you live in, it's beautiful, it's sustains you, and it deserves to be well taken care of. Write a short paragraph of gratitude about your body.

_____
_____
_____
_____
_____
_____
_____

What are some things you can do to take better care of your body?

_____
_____
_____
_____
_____

WATER (CUPS)

◊ ◊ ◊ ◊ ◊ ◊ ◊ ◊

SLEEP (HRS)

◯ ◯ ◯ ◯ ◯ ◯ ◯ ◯

MOOD (FEEL)

☺ ☺ ☺ ☹ ☹ ☺ ☹

EXERCISE (MIN)

FOOD LOG

Day Seven

So far, you have learned how to restore your mindset, be more thankful, remove toxic things from your environment, Spend more time outdoors, drink more water, sleep better, and exercise a little more! WOW! Congratulations! You are making incredible progress in your journey to feeling more like yourself.

Please return to your first few journal entries and remember how that felt! Can you see that you have come a LONG way! You are so brave and committed to this process. Write freely about how you are feeling now vs when you first began. Assess your strengths and be thankful for them.

_____

_____

_____

_____

_____

_____

_____

_____

_____

WATER (CUPS)

⬯ ⬯ ⬯ ⬯ ⬯ ⬯ ⬯ ⬯

_____

SLEEP (HRS)

○ ○ ○ ○ ○ ○ ○ ○ ○

_____

MOOD (FEEL)

☺ ☺ ☺ ☹ ☹ ☺ ☺

_____

EXERCISE (MIN)

_____

FOOD LOG

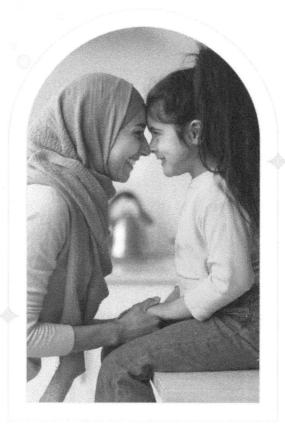

For a mother, eating well is an act of self-love and a gift to her family. She nurtures her body like a cherished garden so she can bloom alongside her children.

The Block Diet

"The food you eat can be either the safest and most powerful form of medicine or the slowest form of poison." - Ann Wigmore.

"Let food be thy medicine, and medicine be thy food." - Hippocrates.

"You are what you eat." - Anthelme Brillat-Savarin.

"Every time you eat or drink, you are either feeding disease or fighting it." - Heather Morgan.

"Health requires healthy food." - Roger Williams.

Hmm, that was different, wasn't it. All these quotes about food and its service to us are inspiring because we live in a time when most of us choose the easy/instant route for everything, including our wellness. But the pillar of truth, that you can simply change the input if you desire a different output, still stands as the safest way to achieve your wellness goals. I want you to be encouraged and know that you have a lot of control over your body, health, and life. When you choose natural solutions, the process may seem slower, but a lot is going on under the surface, and you will you will get there healthfully.

 Most of us dont have questions about what we should be eating but instead, struggle with how to stop eating the foods we know are not serving us, How to stop the cravings for addictive foods, and What to do about our family members who won't come along on our journey. Today, we will talk about all those questions, but first, I will remind you of the main categories of foods and how they help your hormone health.

Yummy Carbs

Carbohydrates are NOT the devil! Phew!, I said it. Carbs have a really bad reputation as fat factories and while there are bits of truth in that it's certainly only true when we overdo them. Your brain, muscles and overall energy needs are powered by carbohydrates. The issue is that we are usually eating processed and simple carbs which don't serve our body well.

Avoid Simple carbs like refined sugars, white flour, and processed (packaged) foods that can cause spikes in blood sugar levels, leading to imbalances in insulin, an essential hormone in regulating blood sugar. Insulin, when out of balance, can also trigger a domino effect on other hormones to get out of balance.

Instead, look for complex carbohydrates in whole grains like quinoa, brown rice, legumes, vegetables, fruits, and some tubers. These foods are rich in fiber, and when you eat them in smaller quantities, they can promote a steady release of insulin and help you feel fuller for longer.

Proteins and Hormone Health

Proteins are the building blocks of every cell that makes up your body. They provide essential amino acids for hormone synthesis and regulate various bodily functions. It's important that we focus on choosing high-quality protein sources, like the proteins from plants. There is a difference between plant-based protein and fake meat, often called meat substitutes. These can often be worse than animal proteins because they often contain ingredients that are highly processed and even ingredients that are strange and hard to pronounce. However, great sources of plant proteins are legumes, nuts, seeds, and even grains like quinoa. Avoid processed meats and high-fat cuts, which can contribute to inflammation and hormonal imbalances. I always encourage people to buy their meat locally at farmers' markets or from nearby farmers if they must continue eating meat.

Additionally, incorporating omega-3 fatty acids from fatty fish like salmon and trout can positively affect hormone health. Omega-3s help reduce inflammation and support brain function, which can indirectly influence hormone regulation.

The idea of "the Block Diet" is simply to make you more aware that everything you eat builds your mind and body. So, choose pieces that give you the structural outcome you desire.

(I've made a table with the top 100 list of foods, and you can check out which hormones they affect and the overall health score. Access it at www.everydaynurse/tools.)

Scrumptious Fats

Fats are necessary in your diet because your body uses fat for hormones, cell membranes, nerves, and other functions in our beautiful bodies, but not all fats are created equal.

When choosing fats to add to your diet, focus on unsaturated fats like avocados, olive oil, coconut oil, fish, nuts, and seeds. Avoid saturated and trans fats like those in fried foods, packaged processed foods, and some "vegetable" derived oils. Instead, emphasize hor-

WEEK 9

mone-positive fats such as those in avocados, nuts, seeds, olive oil, and fatty fish. Intentionally incorporating omega-3 fatty acids from sources like flaxseeds, chia seeds, and walnuts can positively affect hormone health. Omega-3s help reduce inflammation and support hormone balance, which is especially beneficial for women.

So now that you have a reminder of the different sources of nutrition, let's get back to those habits, cravings and social pressure that's often hard to ignore.

Letting go of certain foods is a common struggle that connects us all in a shared journey toward better health. The craving foods we have become addicted to, either physically or emotionally, can feel overpowering, making us feel as though we are at the mercy of our taste buds. It's not just about willpower; it's about understanding the 'why' behind our cravings and patiently untangling ourselves from the addictions towards healthier choices that still satisfy those deep-seated needs for comfort and pleasure. Sometimes, our cravings are a signal from our body about an unmet need, whether it's nutritional, emotional, or physical. Other times, they're simply a habit loop we've fallen into. I often encourage women I consult with to study the food they are craving, look at the nutritional profile of that food, and see what it is offering their body. Sometimes, we are caving micronutrients; sometimes, we have become addicted to certain additives like MSG or other things added to foods to keep us coming back. Breaking that loop means creating new, healthier patterns that fulfill us in ways those old cravings never could.

For many people, healthy food means bland, unseasoned, and unsatisfying. I have experienced this every time I try to order a healthier version of a dish in a restaurant. Sometimes, it's barely even salted. On the journey to health, you need to be sure not just to take away but also add things that make it yummy and fun. Find delicious replica recipes of your favorite dishes without the unhealthy ingredients. Trust me, our life is just as full, fun, and delicious on a primarily plant-based diet.

Then there's the matter of our loved ones who might not be on the same page as us. Trying to make healthier choices can feel lonely while those around us continue with the status quo. But here's where love, patience, and creativity come into play. It's about leading by example, sharing the delicious and nourishing meals that have brought you joy, and finding ways to make this journey inclusive without judgment or pressure. Your journey can inspire, not through words, but through the vibrant energy, health, and happiness that your choices bring into your life.

WEEK 9

Start small. Pick one habit you'd like to change and approach it with understanding and kindness. Why is this food a go-to for you? What healthier choice could satisfy the same need? Remember, it's not about perfection; it's about progress. Celebrate the small victories, like choosing a piece of fruit over a sugary snack or opting for a homemade meal over fast food. These choices add up fast, especially when you stop and acknowledge your successes.

The food is supposed to be absolutely delicious! But remember, you like what you eat, and you eat what you like. Anything you begin to eat consistently, you will begin to like. I hope that encourages you to try new foods you may not initially think to taste good. They will.

Day one

List the top 20 foods you eat most often. If it's fast food, list the menu item.

_____   _____   _____
_____   _____   _____
_____   _____   _____
_____   _____   _____
_____   _____   _____
_____   _____   _____
_____   _____   _____
_____

Assess your list above. Are they convenience-based, comfort foods, or nourishing choices that fuel your body?

_____
_____
_____
_____

What can you do to improve your relationship with food. Make a plan

_____

WATER (CUPS)

○ ○ ○ ○ ○ ○ ○ ○

SLEEP (HRS)

○ ○ ○ ○ ○ ○ ○ ○

_____

MOOD (FEEL)

☺ ☺ ☺ ☹ ☹ ☺ ☺

_____

EXERCISE (MIN) [   ]

_____

FOOD LOG

_____

_____

Day two

Think about the foods you crave the most. What are they, and when do these cravings usually hit?

_____

_____

_____

_____

_____

_____

Do you notice a pattern or a trigger behind these cravings?

_____

_____

_____

_____

_____

If your cravings are unhealthy, make a plan to allow yourself to have that food but regain control of when and how you enjoy it.

_____

_____

_____

_____

_____

_____

_____

when the next craving hits, pause, Drink a glass of water and wait 10 minutes. Then, see if the craving was a sign of dehydration or a moment of stress.

WATER (CUPS)

◊ ◊ ◊ ◊ ◊ ◊ ◊ ◊

SLEEP (HRS)

○ ○ ○ ○ ○ ○ ○ ○

MOOD (FEEL)

☺ ☺ ☺ ☺ ☺ ☺ ☺

EXERCISE (MIN)

FOOD LOG

Day three

Think back to a moment when your emotions led you to eat. Write about it in detail. (What emotions trigger this response, and what foods do you reach for?)

_____

_____

_____

_____

_____

_____

Describe your feelings after you eat based on an emotional response

_____

_____

_____

_____

Look up a healthy new food or recipe you would like to try and write it down. Even reducing the amount of butter or sugar in a recipe is a great start!

_____

_____

_____

_____

_____

_____

WATER (CUPS)

◇ ◇ ◇ ◇ ◇ ◇ ◇ ◇

SLEEP (HRS)

○ ○ ○ ○ ○ ○ ○ ○ ○

MOOD (FEEL)

☺ ☺ ☺ ☹ ☹ ☺ ☺

EXERCISE (MIN) [____]

FOOD LOG

[   ]

Day Four

Think about what you want to achieve with your dietary changes. Is it better health, more energy, improved mood, or something else? Write down your goals and why they're important to you.

_____

_____

_____

_____

_____

_____

_____

Why do you want these goals? What is the deep overarching reason beneath the surface? Dig deep and let it all out.

_____

_____

_____

WATER (CUPS)

◌ ◌ ◌ ◌ ◌ ◌ ◌ ◌

SLEEP (HRS)

◯ ◯ ◯ ◯ ◯ ◯ ◯ ◯

MOOD (FEEL)

☺ ☺ ☺ ☹ ☹ ☺ ☹

EXERCISE (MIN)

FOOD LOG

Go to your pantry and remove ONE thing that should not be in there. It should never return.

Day five

What food changes have you made so far and how does it make you feel?

_____
_____
_____
_____
_____
_____
_____

List 5 things you feel have gone well so far in your transformation journey.

_____
_____
_____
_____
_____
_____

Think of the changes you would like to make in your diet and make a plan to slowly do so.

_____
_____
_____
_____
_____
_____

WATER (CUPS)

○ ○ ○ ○ ○ ○ ○ ○

SLEEP (HRS)

○ ○ ○ ○ ○ ○ ○ ○ ○ ○

MOOD (FEEL)

☺ ☺ ☺ ☹ ☹ ☺ ☺

EXERCISE (MIN)

FOOD LOG

Day Six

Choose one food you crave or eat that you know isn't good for your health. Research and write down its nutritional profile and how it affects your body and hormones.

_____

_____

_____

_____

_____

_____

_____

_____

_____

_____

_____

_____

_____

Think of 7 foods you are thankful for

_____

_____

_____

_____

_____

_____

_____

WATER (CUPS)

SLEEP (HRS)

MOOD (FEEL)

EXERCISE (MIN)

FOOD LOG

Day Seven

Write freely and express gratitude for all the things you are learning. Be thankful for the new things you tried this week. Express gratitude for your dedication to the transformation you are going through.

_____

_____

_____

_____

_____

_____

_____

_____

_____

_____

_____

_____

WATER (CUPS)

⬡ ⬡ ⬡ ⬡ ⬡ ⬡ ⬡ ⬡

SLEEP (HRS)

○ ○ ○ ○ ○ ○ ○ ○

MOOD (FEEL)

☺ ☻ ☺ ☹ ☹ ☺ ☹

EXERCISE (MIN) [   ]

FOOD LOG

[   ]

Step four
Behavior Alteration

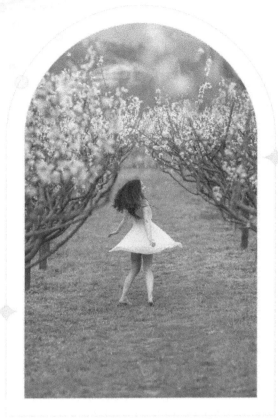

Transformation is the silent unfolding of your heart, where each tear and smile weaves a story so deep, it turns the ordinary into a beautiful story of enduring grace and beauty.

Un-Comfort-Able

There are few things we humans dread more than change. Change is the unknown. Change is uncomfortable. Change means growing pains, even if the expected outcome is positive. It can sometimes feel like a dark tunnel because we don't control the outcome and cannot tell if the change will serve us until we "get there." Change has carried double its dread since becoming a mother because I know that when I change something, I am upsetting the ecosystem of FIVE WHOLE other humans! Something as simple as a hairstyle change for me can have five varied responses ranging from meltdowns about how this person loved the last way I had my hair to excited suggestions that turn into arguments about how I should wear it next. Oh my! While it does not stop us from experiencing life, moving to that new home, or even, yes, changing our hair again next week, change does come with its fair share of apprehension and sometimes subconscious stress.

Change can bring up feelings of resistance, and I would like to give you the tools to over-come that resistance and keep climbing the steep hill despite your internal desire to slide back down to your comfort zone, which hasn't been serving you well. I want you to win. And I know you do, too.

First, you must realize that you are like a rubber band; all your habits, nuances, and thought patterns are just rubber bands, and you have a powerful desire not to be stretched. Every time you get stretched a little, you return to your form as soon as the pressure decreases. It's comfortable but ineffective; you're just lying there out of shape in many ways. Everything you learn seeks to stretch you and give you purpose, to hold concepts together, to tie into something and become purposeful like a friendship bracelet, but you resist it. We all do. Knowing this will help you realize there is war ahead: The new you vs the familiar are about to go head to head. You must stretch yourself out of shape until the rubber band takes a new form until it is so far stretched that it does not spring back as easily into the past.

Expect emotional, physical, and mental resistance. Remember, "intention is always followed by disruption- Myron Golden," but you now have the tools to move forward in spite of the disruption that will surely come. Disruption can be internal or external, So you MUST keep your thoughts positive and keep moving forward no matter what.

You cannot stop learning. You need the momentum of information and shared experiences to keep you moving. The ideas that are changing your life are just the beginning. This journal has been a fantastic tool to help you start your journey. There is a world ahead, and you cannot take it all in one bite, so it's incredible that you have come this far in your journey, are experiencing so many great things, and are starting to recognize yourself again. I LOVE IT FOR YOU! And I want you to keep that positive progress by continuing to learn.

While you learn, you will find many things out there that may sound similar to the things you've implemented and that are working so well for you. I have never been one to fear opposition, and I don't want you to either because truth is not afraid of opposition; it just stands true and will remain. So, as you hear things you are unfamiliar with, do your due diligence, study, and see who is sponsoring the research. If you love reading research papers like I do, ensure that the research was conducted for educational purposes and not by someone biased trying to sell you something. Then, add to or edit parts of your current process as you see fit, but never stop learning.

Another excellent tool to keep moving forward despite the negative pull from your resistance to change is to join a community. Local communities are the absolute best if you have access to them. Join a community of like-minded people who are moving forward and want to live as the best version of themselves and enjoy their children as much as you do. Join a positive army so you can win the war. Negative armies will drag you down, so please be very selective. Once you are in a group surrounded by stories that inspire you and an opportunity to inspire others, this can become a sort of accountability for you. Share your wins and your struggles, and allow the embrace of a supportive community to nurture you when you are down. If you cannot find a local group, consider online groups geared towards your goals. Take an active role in the group and make friends you can talk to regularly that align with your values and goals. Remember, the key is to make sure the person is not a downpour but someone with whom you can grow and make positive progress.

The third tool I think is crucial in any journey is your "WHY ." Why" are you going through all of this change? Is the reason strong enough to keep you going? Certainly, the discomfort of not feeling like yourself and all the symptoms of your imbalance were strong enough to get you to desire a change, but are they stronger than the discomfort of change itself? These are questions you need to ask yourself, and you need to have an honest assessment of where you stand so that you can anticipate your weak points and begin to feel when you need some reinforcement. One way to keep a reminder of the 'Why' is to have a detailed journal documenting your journey. Whenever you need a reminder, scroll back to the early days and look at yourself to see how far you have come. Not only will you be amazed at the strides you've made, but you will also be convinced that there is no going back!

WEEK 10

At EverydayNurse.com, you will find additional tools that can support your change, including communities and groups you can join, as well as blogs and articles from myself and other guest authors that will continue to move you in a positive direction.

Day one

Try to recall your last significant change; how did you feel about it?

_____

_____

_____

_____

_____

_____

_____

Did you feel like you had a choice in any of it? Explain

_____

_____

_____

_____

_____

_____

WATER (CUPS)

〇 〇 〇 〇 〇 〇 〇 〇

How do you want to choose to view change moving
forward?

SLEEP (HRS)

〇 〇 〇 〇 〇 〇 〇 〇

_____

MOOD (FEEL)

😊 🙂 😐 🙁 😢 😁 😐

_____

EXERCISE (MIN)

_____

FOOD LOG

_____

Day two

What are some of your reasons for resisting change? List your top 3

_____

_____

_____

_____

_____

_____

_____

_____

Think, pray, and write out some possible solutions for each of the above.

_____

_____

_____

_____

_____

_____

WATER (CUPS)

◊ ◊ ◊ ◊ ◊ ◊ ◊ ◊

SLEEP (HRS)

○ ○ ○ ○ ○ ○ ○ ○

MOOD (FEEL)

☺ ☺ ☺ ☹ ☹ ☺ ☺

EXERCISE (MIN)

FOOD LOG

Dedicate 30 minutes to learning something related to your goals for change. It could be a podcast, an article, or a chapter in a book.

Day three

Describe YOU. The new you, the true you, with some of those beautiful elements you recall from the past, but more mature, calm, more beautiful with age, more resilient, more valuable like fine crisp wine. Answer the Following questions about her... (the true you)

What does she look like
_____
_____
_____

What does she wear
_____
_____
_____

What does she like to eat?
_____
_____
_____

Who does she hang out with
_____
_____
_____

WATER (CUPS)

○ ○ ○ ○ ○ ○ ○ ○

SLEEP (HRS)

○ ○ ○ ○ ○ ○ ○ ○

How does she feel about herself?
_____
_____
_____
_____
_____

MOOD (FEEL)

☺ ☺ ☺ ☹ ☹ ☺ ☺

EXERCISE (MIN) [   ]

FOOD LOG

[   ]

Day Four

Because the material in this book was compressed to fit the journal format, there is a wealth of information out there. What are you excited to learn more about?

_____

_____

_____

_____

_____

_____

What do you feel are your strong points in the journey so far?

_____

_____

_____

_____

_____

_____

_____

Make a plan to strengthen your weak points.

_____

_____

_____

_____

_____

_____

WATER (CUPS)

○ ○ ○ ○ ○ ○ ○ ○

SLEEP (HRS)

○ ○ ○ ○ ○ ○ ○ ○ ○

MOOD (FEEL)

☺ ☺ ☺ ☹ ☹ ☺ ☺

EXERCISE (MIN)

FOOD LOG

Day five

Do you have a supportive community. Describe it. If not, describe your desired community and then find it

_____

_____

_____

_____

_____

_____

Has your community been serving you and bringing you growth

_____

_____

_____

_____

_____

_____

_____

_____

WATER (CUPS)

◊ ◊ ◊ ◊ ◊ ◊ ◊ ◊

Are there any communities/ associations you must separate from to move forward? explain then DO IT

SLEEP (HRS)

○ ○ ○ ○ ○ ○ ○ ○ ○

_____

MOOD (FEEL)

☺ ☺ ☺ ☹ ☹ ☺ ☺

_____

EXERCISE (MIN) [   ]

_____

FOOD LOG

_____

Join growth communities (find suggestions at www.EverydayNurse.com/tools)

Day Six

What is your WHY– the reason you decided to go through this journey? Search deep within you, Write it out, and state every detail.

_____

_____

_____

_____

_____

_____

_____

_____

_____

_____

_____

_____

_____

_____

_____

_____

WATER (CUPS)

⬠ ⬠ ⬠ ⬠ ⬠ ⬠ ⬠ ⬠

SLEEP (HRS)

◯ ◯ ◯ ◯ ◯ ◯ ◯ ◯

MOOD (FEEL)

☺ ☺ ☺ ☹ ☹ ☺ ☺

EXERCISE (MIN)

FOOD LOG

If you are struggling and need more help please reach out or seek proffessional help

Day Seven

Gratitude Day! Write out your gratitude. Free flow and fill the page!

_____

_____

_____

_____

_____

_____

_____

_____

_____

_____

_____

_____

_____

_____

WATER (CUPS)

◊ ◊ ◊ ◊ ◊ ◊ ◊ ◊

SLEEP (HRS)

○ ○ ○ ○ ○ ○ ○ ○

MOOD (FEEL)

☺ ☺ ☺ ☹ ☹ ☺ ☺

EXERCISE (MIN)

FOOD LOG

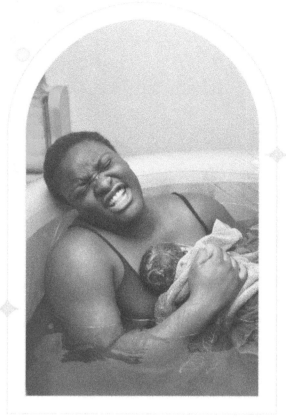

Bravery is facing storms with a gentle smile, transforming fear into pathways of strength, and weaving a legacy of courage and love that resonates through time.

It's Your Turn.
The next chapter is your
story, how you got here, who
you are, and who you are
becoming.

Celebrate your wins, Let go of
the losses, appreciate the
journey, and best of all, Look
ahead to a beautiful
tomorrow.

YOU. CAN. DO. THIS.

A New Start

_____

_____

_____

_____

_____

_____

_____

_____

_____

_____

_____

_____

_____

_____

_____

_____

_____

_____

_____

WEEK 11

WEEK 11

Day one

What does holistic health mean to you? How do you currently incorporate a holistic approach to wellness in your life?

_____

_____

_____

_____

_____

_____

_____

_____

Identify areas where you feel strong and areas that might need more attention (physical, emotional, mental, and spiritual health).

_____

_____

_____

_____

_____

_____

WATER (CUPS)

○ ○ ○ ○ ○ ○ ○ ○ ○

SLEEP (HRS)

○ ○ ○ ○ ○ ○ ○ ○ ○

Think of 3 emotions you are thankful for

MOOD (FEEL)

☺ ☺ ☺ ☹ ☹ ☺ ☺

_____

EXERCISE (MIN) [   ]

_____

FOOD LOG

_____

Day two

Have you experienced the benefits of a natural remedy or holistic practice (e.g., herbal teas, lifestyle changes, breathing techniques)? Describe the experience and the effects it had on your well-being.

_____

_____

_____

_____

_____

_____

_____

_____

Research a natural remedy or holistic practice that addresses your current health concern or goal. Write your findings below.

_____

_____

_____

_____

WATER (CUPS)

◊ ◊ ◊ ◊ ◊ ◊ ◊ ◊

SLEEP (HRS)

○ ○ ○ ○ ○ ○ ○ ○

MOOD (FEEL)

☺ ☺ ☺ ☹ ☹ ☺ ☹

EXERCISE (MIN)

FOOD LOG

Day three

How does your current community (family, friends, online groups) support or hinder your wellness goals?

_____

_____

_____

_____

_____

How well do you feel you understand your body's signals? Are there signals or symptoms you've ignored? list them below and make a plan to address them

_____

_____

_____

_____

_____

_____

WATER (CUPS)

◌ ◌ ◌ ◌ ◌ ◌ ◌ ◌

SLEEP (HRS)

◯ ◯ ◯ ◯ ◯ ◯ ◯ ◯

MOOD (FEEL)

☺ ☺ ☺ ☹ ☹ ☺ ☺

EXERCISE (MIN)

FOOD LOG

Day Four

Take a moment to Imagine your life transformed by fully embracing holistic health. What does this look like regarding your daily habits, how you feel physically and emotionally, and how are your relationships affected? You should write it out as if you are fully there right now.

_____
_____
_____
_____
_____
_____
_____
_____
_____
_____
_____
_____
_____
_____

WATER (CUPS)

◊ ◊ ◊ ◊ ◊ ◊ ◊ ◊

SLEEP (HRS)

○ ○ ○ ○ ○ ○ ○ ○ ○

MOOD (FEEL)

☺ ☺ ☺ ☹ ☹ ☺ ☹

EXERCISE (MIN)

FOOD LOG

If your answer above represents your desire, say a prayer about it.

Day five

Think about your childhood. What did you feel called to do at an early age? Who did you want to become? I do not mean the career choices that children are so often steered into, but the girl who had a cause she wanted to fight for or a people group she wanted to serve. Please write out that call and let it all out.

_____

_____

_____

_____

_____

_____

_____

_____

_____

_____

_____

_____

_____

WATER (CUPS)

◊ ◊ ◊ ◊ ◊ ◊ ◊ ◊

SLEEP (HRS)

○ ○ ○ ○ ○ ○ ○ ○ ○

MOOD (FEEL)

☺ ☺ ☺ ☺ ☺ ☺ ☺

EXERCISE (MIN)

FOOD LOG

It's never too late. You are still here. Take a step towards your dream today...just a step.

Day Six

How are you feeling about your mental health these days?

_____

_____

_____

_____

_____

_____

_____

Review earlier chapters and how you felt as you read and went through the journal portion. Do you feel like you are the same person? Explain.

_____

_____

_____

_____

_____

_____

_____

WATER (CUPS)

⬭ ⬭ ⬭ ⬭ ⬭ ⬭ ⬭ ⬭

SLEEP (HRS)

◯ ◯ ◯ ◯ ◯ ◯ ◯ ◯

MOOD (FEEL)

☺ ☹ ☺ ☹ ☹ ☺ ☹

EXERCISE (MIN)

FOOD LOG

Do you feel like you need help finding your purpose? If you do, please visit EverydayNurse.com/tools and look for the ' finding purpose tool kit'. Cheers to you living in your purpose.

Day Seven

Identify 12 people in your life that you are grateful for. Make a note, Write, a letter, call or text to let them know you appreciate them.

_____

_____

_____

_____

_____

_____

_____

_____

_____

Think about your favorite spot in nature and describe it

_____

_____

_____

_____

WATER (CUPS)

⬠ ⬠ ⬠ ⬠ ⬠ ⬠ ⬠ ⬠

SLEEP (HRS)

○ ○ ○ ○ ○ ○ ○ ○

MOOD (FEEL)

☺ ☺ ☺ ☹ ☹ ☺ ☺

EXERCISE (MIN) [   ]

FOOD LOG

[   ]

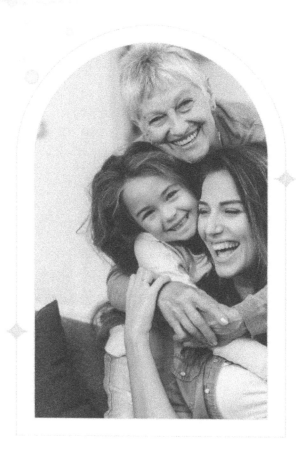

Motherhood is the endless embrace of love and sacrifice

Plant Powered Wellness

Sometimes, we all need a little help. And it's ok. Depending on our past experiences, we sometimes struggle to ask for help, but I will offer you lots of help on this journey to freedom. Unfortunately, I cannot provide some of the excellent sauna sessions and massages I enjoyed during my transformation experience. I highly recommend you find some of those services around you. It's so great to relax, detoxify, and be pampered every now and again. In my other book, "Prevention is Cheaper Than Cure," I challenge the norm of trying to save money on the front end by eating less healthy options or not engaging in health-boosting activities to save a dollar, and end up spending ten times that amount on health challenges that come because of neglecting our wellness. So prevention is indeed cheaper, girl; go get that massage.

Now that I've convinced you to get a spa date set to release some of that stress let's talk about some of the herbs which are widely used to aid women's wellness. Research the herbs and speak to your healthcare provider if needed.

Wild Yam

The very first one I used in my journey, which is worthy of mention, is wild yam. I have used wild yam powder from Amazon and the root pieces that I steeped into tea, and I have also used it in cream form. Wild yam cream is a natural plant-based alternative to chemical-based progesterone creams. Wild yams are said to have an element that helps with progesterone boosting and is also said to have anti-inflammatory properties. It has been absolutely incredible for some women who have used wild yam cream and me. I loved the ease of use and knowing that no toxic ingredients were present in the creams I used. I've only used two brands of creams (Both of which I have made available on the storefront at www.EverydayNurse.com/store).

Red Raspberry leaves

I personally enjoy the golden raspberries better than the red ones, but the red raspberries are said to have the good stuff in their leaves. I typically steep the leaves and sometimes add some lemon and a bit of honey, or just have it plain and sip away. I've even chilled it in batches and had it in place of water throughout my day.

WEEK 12

Chamomile Tea

Chamomile may not be on your typical hormone health herb list, but I have used it to help me calm down when I have been a bit high-strung and anxious, and as an added bonus, it tends to help me sleep sweetly.

Maca

There is a running joke that my second child is a Maca baby. Ehem... well, Maca can have side effects like increasing your libido, and it certainly did for me. Yet, it may be a great herb to add to your hormone reset regimen. I used to add it to my smoothies and baked goods, and if I did not add too much, I could barely even taste its presence.

Red clover

Another herb I used in my tea mixes was red clover, which has an earthy taste similar to red raspberry leaves. While I cannot say I ever felt an immediate difference from drinking red clover leaf tea, it was part of my regimen, and I trust that I reaped its benefits.

There are so many more herbs and teas, tinctures, and concoctions, so while you may find yourself diving into that world, I do want you to remain careful and vigilant and do your due diligence. Remember that simple is best for your body and what you put in or on it.

Even though you are at the end of this 12-week journey, if you could benefit from going through it again, please, please do. Just start over and fill everything out in a notebook. The second or third time is when it may set in for you. This is not a race, and your habits and thought patterns may need another round of washing, so don't be shy about turning the pages back to one. If you may benefit from going through the program with other like-minded women in the community, I welcome you to join the next 12-week 'Hormone Reset Pathway' program. You will find that information and many more tools you can use on your journey on www.EverydayNurse.com or scan the QR code below.

Scan me

Day one

Herbs and supplements are not everyone's cup of tea. A quick look at the polarizing information on the internet will clarify that. What are your thoughts on herbs, supplements, and other natural aids for health

_____

_____

_____

_____

_____

_____

Which Herbs, supplements or remedies have you tried with success?

_____

_____

_____

_____

_____

_____

WATER (CUPS)

◇ ◇ ◇ ◇ ◇ ◇ ◇ ◇

SLEEP (HRS)

○ ○ ○ ○ ○ ○ ○ ○

MOOD (FEEL)

☺ ☺ ☺ ☹ ☹ ☺ ☺

EXERCISE (MIN)

FOOD LOG

Day two

How is your exercise Routine going? What have you learned about yourself, your strength and discipline through exercise?

_____

_____

_____

_____

_____

_____

_____

How do you feel about your body now? Describe your energy levels and your feelings about your physical body

_____

_____

_____

_____

_____

WATER (CUPS)

◇ ◇ ◇ ◇ ◇ ◇ ◇ ◇

SLEEP (HRS)

○ ○ ○ ○ ○ ○ ○ ○

MOOD (FEEL)

☺ ☺ ☺ ☹ ☹ ☺ ☺

EXERCISE (MIN)

FOOD LOG

Day Three

Think back to who you were in Week 1. What mindset shifts have you experienced in the last 12 weeks?

_____

_____

_____

_____

_____

_____

_____

_____

What are some new experiences you have enjoyed because of your mindset shift?

_____

_____

_____

_____

_____

_____

WATER (CUPS)

◌ ◌ ◌ ◌ ◌ ◌ ◌ ◌

Share 5 things you are thankful for

SLEEP (HRS)

○ ○ ○ ○ ○ ○ ○ ○

_____

MOOD (FEEL)

☺ ☹ ☺ ☹ ☹ ☺ ☺

_____

EXERCISE (MIN) [   ]

_____

FOOD LOG

_____

_____

Day Four

Write down your most significant transformation in the last 12 weeks. Close your eyes for a few minutes and really search your heart for this one.

_____
_____
_____
_____
_____
_____
_____
_____

Have you been celebrating your wins? it's important to do so!
Describe the ultimate celebration You will have when you finish this program at the end of this week.

_____
_____
_____
_____
_____

List 5 WINS you are thankful for.

WATER (CUPS)
◊ ◊ ◊ ◊ ◊ ◊ ◊ ◊

SLEEP (HRS)
○ ○ ○ ○ ○ ○ ○

MOOD (FEEL)
☺ ☺ ☺ ☹ ☹ ☺ ☺

EXERCISE (MIN)

FOOD LOG

Day five

What is one new habit that has become a natural part of your life? Write the details about how you achieved that. (You can use the same strategy in areas where you may be struggling.)

_____

_____

_____

_____

_____

Out of all the changes you have been making with your time outdoors, diet, exercise, water intake, mindset, sleep habits, and all, which one was the easiest for you to master and why?

_____

_____

_____

_____

Have your close relationships improved? Explain

_____

_____

_____

_____

_____

WATER (CUPS)

◊ ◊ ◊ ◊ ◊ ◊ ◊ ◊

SLEEP (HRS)

○ ○ ○ ○ ○ ○ ○ ○

MOOD (FEEL)

☺ ☺ ☺ ☹ ☹ ☺ ☹

EXERCISE (MIN)

FOOD LOG

Day Six

It's your last week journaling in this program. How do you feel about that? (Vent)

_____

_____

_____

_____

_____

_____

What structures have you established to help you continue in the right direction?

_____

_____

_____

_____

_____

_____

What changes are you looking forward to making a part of your forever?

_____

_____

_____

_____

_____

_____

_____

WATER (CUPS)

◊ ◊ ◊ ◊ ◊ ◊ ◊ ◊

SLEEP (HRS)

○ ○ ○ ○ ○ ○ ○ ○

MOOD (FEEL)

☺ ☺ ☺ ☹ ☹ ☺ ☺

EXERCISE (MIN)

FOOD LOG

Day Seven

I am sad to be writing the last page of this wellness journal. It's been my absolute pleasure to come along and guide you through this journey. Thank you for trusting me to help you achieve wellness. Thank you for gathering the courage to come this far! You are INCREDIBLE! I want you to know that you are precious and deeply loved by your Creator and community. Keep striving to grow; Water your tender habits until they bud and blossom.

Today, write a letter to God. Pour out your heart to Him, let Him fill your mind, and renew your body.

_____

_____

_____

_____

_____

_____

_____

_____

_____

_____

_____

WATER (CUPS)

○ ○ ○ ○ ○ ○ ○ ○

SLEEP (HRS)

○ ○ ○ ○ ○ ○ ○ ○

MOOD (FEEL)

☺ ☺ ☺ ☺ ☺ ☺ ☺

EXERCISE (MIN)

FOOD LOG

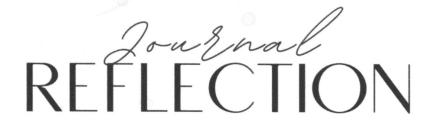

Journal REFLECTION

Q1 What are you most proud of after completing this book?

....

....

....

....

Would you recommend it to a friend? **Q2**

....

....

....

....

Q3

How may we further help you?

....

....

....

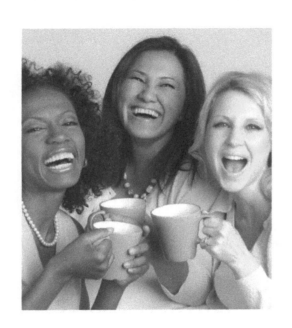

NEED MORE INSIGHT & SUPPORT?

Scan me

Would you like more professional or community support?
Do you want to keep going and achieve your ideal wellness?
We are here to help.
Visit www.EverydayNurse.com

www.ingramcontent.com/pod-product-compliance
Lightning Source LLC
LaVergne TN
LVHW081244070425
807931LV00011B/81